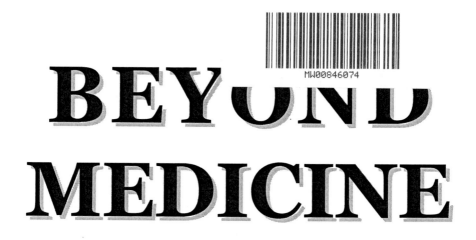

BEYOND MEDICINE

6 ELEMENTS OF HEALING

LOVE
PRAYER
HUMOR
TOUCH
MUSIC
PETS

...based on experiences with ARDS
(Acute Respiratory Distress Syndrome)
and other critical illnesses

STEPHEN R. YARNALL, MD

First Edition

Thornton Publishing Inc.
17011 Lincoln Ave. #408
Parker, CO 80134

303-794-8888

BooksToBelieveIn.com

Proudly printed in the United States of America
ISBN: 0-9670242-8-5

Readers' Comments

·   I highly recommend Dr. Yarnall's gripping story to you. Journey to the edge of life with Steve and then return to a fuller life with him. You will find the trip to be an exciting ride you will never forget.

Lester R. Sauvage, M.D.
Cardiovascular Surgeon
Founder, The Hope Heart Institute
Author of "The Open Heart"

·   From the perspective of patients and family members, Dr. Yarnall reveals the sources of strength that ordinary people can draw upon when faced with a catastrophic illness.

John Hansen-Flaschen, M.D.
Professor of Medicine& Chief of Pulmonary,
Allergy and Critical Care Division
University of Pennsylvania School of Medicine

·   At a time when medical technology seems to be the answer in life threatening illnesses, you bring us back to the realization that it is not just high-tech, but also family and community support ... You have touched something vital in the American way of thinking ...whatever it is, it's beyond medicine.

Noel Tiano, ThD.
Former Chaplain at Washoe Medical Center

·   Not only are you trying to teach the world about Acute Respiratory Distress Syndrome - (which I had not heard of prior to reading your book), but you are presenting a theory of consciousness which far transcends ARDS.

Maralyn Chase, State Representative
32nd Legislative District, State of Washington

·   This book is a magnificent revelation about a little-known disease - ARDS. The stories of sheer courage of ARDS patients makes it difficult to put this book down once started. This book is a "must read" for everyone.

Alexander Rayshich,   77 year old retired Engineer

·   This book is so good that I'm sending a copy to each of our Board Members.

Jeannette Dunn, Director
Foundation for Care Management

This is a wonderful, helpful book for the critically ill patient, family and friends. Healthy readers can see what the patient is REALLY going through. I know since I was a 42-year old ARDS patient following surgery for a stomach ulcer in April, 2000.

Nancy Lackemacher
Retired Budget Analyst
Sacramento, California

DEDICATIONS AND ACKNOWLEDGEMENTS

To my wife, Lynn, my cheerleader, prayer leader and constant companion "in sickness and in health.";

> *To my family who spent many days and nights praying by my bedside: Tom, Mary, Matthew Tenzin, Bob, David, Gail, Kim, Mike, Terry, Jeanie, Nancy, David S, Trudy, Myra, Lindsay, Jaylinn, Terri, Barbara and Tom R;*

To my many friends and patients whose love, prayers, and encouragement led me to a second life;

> *To my life-saving physician and now friend, Dr. Bob Watson, and to all the physicians, nurses and staff at Washoe Medical Center;*

To Dr. Len Hudson and his many helpers (MD, RN, RT, OT, PT, ST, "DT" – dog therapy) at Seattle's Harborview Medical Center.

> *To Dr. David Heard and his staff who rehabilitated me so well at Northwest Hospital in Seattle.*

To countless prayer groups and individuals around the world who gave me a new outlook on prayer;

> *To Joel Goodman, Margie Ingram and the HUMOR PROJECT, the Seattle Seafair Clowns, and all who brought and kept humor in my life;*

To all those who contributed their stories, especially Meg Tapucol-Provo and Eileen Zacharias;

> *To my editors and text coordinators: Erin Audley and June Cornett;*

To E.J. Thornton, who patiently worked with me to publish "Beyond Medicine"; and

> *To you and each of my readers who trusted that they would find information, inspiration and humor in Beyond Medicine, may these words and bring you love and peace and allow you to find powers of healing beyond medicine.*

Foreword

Lester R. Sauvage, MD
Founder, The Hope Heart Institute

When you read Dr. Yarnall's exceptional book, *Beyond Medicine,* be prepared for a journey that may change your life. It did his. Steve has been where few have gone. His experiences have reshaped his life in mysterious ways that he precisely describes in some areas by beautiful prose and in others through feelings because there are no adequate words.

Steve tells us that we have a future beyond this life and that it can be wonderful. He didn't have to write this book, but I believe that an inner, holy power lead him by the hand to do so. This is a remarkable book by a remarkable physician who is now not afraid to say that there is more to life than a black nothing at the end.

I find Steve's book to be full of hope for what can lie beyond for all of us. This book is a story of exciting adventure into the largely unknown. It will challenge your mind to open wide and consider that you are far more than mere matter, so much more.

I highly recommend Dr. Yarnall's gripping story to you. Journey to the edge of life with Steve and then return to a fuller life with him. You will find the trip to be an exciting ride you will never forget.

Foreword

John Hansen-Flaschen, M.D.
Professor of Medicine
Chief, Pulmonary, Allergy and Critical Care Division
University of Pennsylvania School of Medicine

The diagnosis, "acute respiratory distress syndrome" (ARDS), the medical disorder that forms the backbone of this book, did not exist before the advent of new, life supporting medical technologies just a few years ago.

ARDS is an acute lung injury of such severity that mechanical ventilation is required to prevent imminent death from respiratory failure. For reasons that are still not well understood, many severe but otherwise seemingly unrelated conditions, including major trauma, pneumonia, complications of surgery and sepsis, sometimes lead down a common, final pathway to acute respiratory distress. Before the development of mechanical ventilators for long-term life support in the mid-1960s, everyone who developed respiratory failure from any of these conditions simply suffocated and died. Imagine the experience of the first doctors and nurses who discovered that some patients could recover from acute respiratory failure if ventilation and other vital bodily functions are supported by intensive medical care until healing can occur.

Over the past several decades since the first bold experiments with prolonged mechanical ventilation for respiratory failure, survival for victims of ARDS has improved dramatically. Today, more that 60% of adults afflicted by this devastating disorder recover and leave the hospital alive. Some require life support for only a few days and are able to return home in as little as 10 to 14 days. Others remain entirely dependent for survival on mechanical ventilation, intravenous medications, tube feedings and continuous nursing care for 2 to 3 months or longer. Most remember little or nothing of their experience in the hospital until rehabilitation is well underway. However, family members and close friends remember their crisis well. Survivors and family members alike remember the long, challenging struggle to regain physical and emotional independence after the acute phase of ARDS is over.

Stephen R. Yarnall, M.D., the author of <u>Beyond</u> <u>Medicine,</u> is a practicing cardiologist and is himself a survivor of severe, prolonged ARDS. Dr. Yarnall describes his own experience and that of others who survived ARDS, and some who did not survive. Several moving stories are told in the first person. From the perspective of patients and family members, Dr. Yarnall reveals the sources of strength that ordinary people can draw upon when faced with a catastrophic illness.

This book is for people who wonder what lessons can be learned from personal adversity and for all those who have survived and persevered after ARDS or other life-threatening illness. Families and friends of survivors and of the many who expire will also find information and comfort in <u>Beyond</u> <u>Medicine.</u>

Here are several references you might find useful.

Abrahm J, **Hansen-Flaschen J**. Hospice care for patients with advanced lung disease. *Chest* 121:220-9, 2002.

Hansen-Flaschen J. Dyspnea in the ventilated patient: a call for patient-centered mechanical ventilation. *Respiratory Care* 45:1460-1464, 2000.

Sullivan DJ, **Hansen-Flaschen J**. Termination of life support after major trauma. *Surg Clinics of North America.*80:1055-1066, 2000.

Hansen-Flaschen J. What is wrong here? Request for immediate withdrawal of mechanical ventilation. <u>End of Life Pearls</u>. Edited by JE Heffner and I Byock. Philadelphia, Hanley & Belfus, Inc. pp.25-27, 2002.

Hansen-Flaschen J. Advanced Lung Disease: palliation and terminal care. *Clinics in Chest Medicine* 18:645-55, 1977.

Foreword
Noel Tiano, ThD.
Former Chaplain at Washoe Medical Center

I really congratulate you for addressing "Prayer" and "Love" not from one having a "religious" agenda, but from one who has had a life-changing experience. It is so refreshing! The issues you raise may indeed be subjective and 'touchy-feely' and not necessarily "evidence-based" but how can one argue against testimonies benefiting (instead of harming) others? Nowadays, we often use "narratives" as integral components of program evaluations. Although I must say that prayer can be harmful in public situations where the leader discriminates other faith traditions, or uses prayer to 'sermonize'.

You write with such clarity and simplicity. I wouldn't have guessed you were an M.D. if you hadn't been a patient I visited at Washoe Medical Center. I like your idea of our spirit growing as we grow. What a concept!

The areas that really struck a chord in me are the following:

Your son, Thomas', very poignant questions — regarding the basis of your "God" talk and transformation. I hear you saying that you are in the process of coming to terms with your faith (reinterpreting?) through your Quaker tradition, early familiar prayers, and similar experiences with others. And to be sure, there are more unanswered questions. I just think it is so profound that you showed your vulnerability and would hope that this section would be alluded to in the preface or introduction because it helps readers know where you are coming from.

Prayer as a mystery - I'm reminded of a similar statement from Kirkegaard which runs something like, 'Life is a mystery to be lived, not a problem to be solved.'

Your observation that **strength and number of prayers is fundamental**. Perhaps God really intended humans to learn the art of praying together — individually or in community, across time and space.

In your section on "Love", I would argue against viewing a God in the Old Testament as "judgmental, rule-making," etc. because in Noah's case, God waited over 100 years for people to repent and yet they refused. There was God's patience on the Israelites, as well as loving kindness, compassion, and mercy e.g. in the Book of Psalms, etc. How the prophets wrote and interpreted God's actions may be something else.

Expanding hope: I wholeheartedly agree about the value of hope, and the search for a cure or miracle. In your case, it was the collective hope from your family and friends and one particular physician. Hope is a very powerful medicine. As it has often been said, Faith (related to hope) can move mountains. Nevertheless, for others who are terminally ill or actively dying, **hope can be reframed** to have better quality of life during the last months or year(s), have better pain management, hope for closure/ forgiveness/ restoration, hope for fewer bills, hope for one last cruise, hope to write or videotape ones memoirs. And oftentimes these deaths are not due to lack of prayer, or faith, and should not be construed as defeat on the part of providers, but rather is a given — life-death-life is a continuum. After all in the Christian tradition, Jesus was born, he suffered, died and rose again. Sometimes even death can be healing.

At a time when medical technology seems to be the answer to life-threatening illnesses, you bring us back to the realization that it is not just hi-tech, but also family & community support (both local and global), and faith (love, hope, resilience, etc.). You have touched something so vital in the American way of thinking. We may be coming full circle where curing and caring, science and beliefs are becoming more (re)integrated... Whatever it is, it's "beyond medicine"!

******

TABLE of CONTENTS

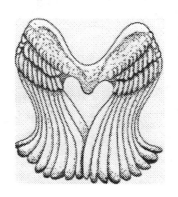

PREFACE – BEYOND MEDICINE

"We have the same final exam this year as last year – only the answers have changed."
Medical School Professor, University of Rochester, 1958

The Answers Keep Changing

Since antiquity, models of medicine have been evolving along a number of pathways. Each new stage is born from knowledge that was one step beyond the current medicine of the day. What is beyond medicine today may be more accepted as part of tomorrow's medicine. ARDS (Acute Respiratory Distress Syndrome) and other critical diseases may be affected by elements of healing often not accepted as part of current medical practice.

As a physician with ARDS I experienced healing forces often considered beyond medicine.

What is ARDS?

ARDS is a mysterious and devastating disease, formerly considered an "Adult" malady, but it affects children also. ARDS has a mortality rate of 30-50% and affects over 150,000 Americans each year. ARDS kills about 75,000 U.S. citizens yearly. About the same number of people die in automobile accidents each year and about the same number of women die from breast cancer each year, yet ARDS is largely unknown to most people and possibly to many doctors.

Prior to my illness, I knew ARDS as "Stiff lung disease" or "White-out of the lung" (based on the fluid in the lung making it opaque – white – on the Chest X-ray). As a practicing physician, I knew enough to call a Lung Specialist, and I knew that these patients usually died. As you will see, ARDS is more than a "Respiratory" disease. As indicated by the word "Syndrome", ARDS is several problems put together. I experienced almost all of those problems with

ARDS, following a 30-foot fall from a ski lift on January 28, 2000. My survival against overwhelming odds was termed a "miracle".

So many people have called me a "Miracle Man" that I have finally come to understand what they mean: It is a miracle that I am alive and back in the practice of medicine. **A miracle is an event that is extremely unlikely in a given circumstance**.

What are "Medical Miracles"?

Since miracles are unpredictable outcomes, miracles are outside the scope of "Evidence-based medicine". Yet, careful observations and analysis of individual cases may lead to treatment guidelines for future patients and may generate testable hypotheses. If a miracle contradicts our understanding of natural laws we are challenged to examine and extend these "laws" – not to reject the miracle.

Where the doctors feel there is little or no chance of recovery, this may be due to lack of physician knowledge or lack of data. But when a patient has a good outcome after being given a "no chance" diagnosis, we may comfortably call this a miracle. Bernie Siegel, M.D. has written about exceptional cancer patients who have outcomes far better than predicted. It appears that miracles can happen in cancer, ARDS, or any disease. Perhaps the elements of healing b*eyond medicine* are the same in all critical disease processes.

Miracles do not refute the laws of science but call us to look for new explanations beyond our current range of knowledge. Paradigm shifts in medicine start with awareness of observations that do not fit existing models.

More attention and studies should be directed at Love, Prayer, Touch, Humor, Music and Pets as separate but interacting *elements of healing*, which may, in some cases, lead to miracles.

I do not give myself credit for producing miracles, but, rather, see myself as the beneficiary of miracles. It is in that sense that I am a "Miracle Man".

What Will I Get From This Book?

BEYOND MEDICINE is relevant, interesting and meant to be read ... not just filed for reference.

As a physician I must note that there are times when life is over for the brain-body as it has been, and a time comes for that person to move on. "Hope" at that point can be directed towards that "Great Unknown" which follows.

While recognizing that you may die prematurely in spite of the best medical care, *BEYOND MEDICINE offers* hopefulness not helplessness. This is NOT a book about the medical details of how to treat ARDS. It is a book about how families and friends can take action on behalf of their loved ones with ARDS or any life-threatening disease - heart, cancer, stroke or other. *BEYOND MEDICINE* is a book about helping miracles happen.

Through my experiences and those of others, you will learn methods and tools beyond medicine to help yourself and others in dealing with a medical crisis wherever you may encounter it.

BEYOND MEDICINE is meant to be as much fun for you to read as it was for me to write. I believe in the "Play Theory of Learning" - which believes changes in thinking, feeling and doing occur most effectively when the mind is in a playful mode. Just as children and pets learn from play, so do adults. I hope you enjoy experiences of "Ah Ha!" and "Ha Ha!" as well as "Ho Ho!" along with a few "Oh Oh's", examining your own life in relation to the stories. We learn and are motivated more from stories than from statistics.

Beyond the excellent Medical care I received, six elements of healing stand out in my ARDS experience: **Love, Prayer, Humor, Touch, Music and Pets**. There may be other elements for you and your family and friends when you encounter a crisis, as you surely will at some time in your life. These true stories give hope to all who are facing high odds against recovery. It has been said, "There are no hopeless situations - only situations where people give up hope".

Stephen R. Yarnall, M.D.
Edmonds, Washington
June 26, 2002

I MY NEAR-DEATH EXPERIENCE WITH ARDS

January 28, 2000 marks the beginning of the story of my near-death experience following a ski-lift accident. Since I was unconscious from the start of this story, I had to rely on what I was told and what was recorded regarding my ARDS. The email records sent almost daily from my wife Lynn, and other family members to a list of over fifty friends and family provided the basis of this chapter.

I went through copies of email records spanning the ninety-two days of my hospitalization and subsequent days of home care. This description from a family perspective amazed me about the miracle of my survival. I divided this chapter into three hospital periods followed by my homecare. Included are reflections on my near death experience by my son Robert.

This section starts with Lynn's account summarizing my hospitalization and her feelings. Following that are edited excerpts from email records from day 2 and after,"beating the odds in Reno."

BEATING THE ODDS IN RENO – Days 1-34

How it all began – Lynn's Account

After a vigorous first ski run we jumped on the chairlift for our second run of the day at Mt. Rose, near Reno, Nevada. For a 66-year old cardiologist, Steve was in pretty good shape. No one can say if what happened next was due to his fatigue, the altitude, dehydration, a drop in blood pressure from sitting still, falling asleep or whatever - but about 100 yards away from the start of the lift, he fainted, had seizure-like movements and fell out of the chairlift. He dropped about 30 feet and miraculously broke no bones. He did, however, hit his head, right arm and chest and bruised his lung.

There was nothing I could do in my state of panic except ride to the top and ski down - which I did without stopping. When I arrived, a doctor who just happened to be skiing by was caring for Steve. The ski patrol had also arrived and were giving him oxygen. They put a neck brace on him before loading him on a toboggan. Steve was breathing but unconscious, with no response as I cried out, "Steve…Steve…can you hear me?"

Tears flowed and I felt helpless, watching him being taken down the slope to a helicopter pad. As they lifted his stretcher into the "bird" to fly him to Washoe Medical Center in Reno, I had a sick feeling in my stomach and an empty feeling in my heart. Was I losing my dear husband?

It was a lonely and scary drive back to Reno. But when I arrived at Washoe the nurses brought me the good news that Steve woke up and had read his own ECG! He was to have a scan to evaluate head and chest injuries. While in the scanner he apparently vomited and had a seizure. Then he was intubated for a low blood oxygen level. To keep him from fighting the ventilator he was sedated and given muscle-paralyzing medicine. He was then moved to the ICU.

Communicating With Family and Friends

My next step was to call family members in Washington, Michigan and New York to let them know that Steve was injured and critically ill. Family members started arriving the very next day. My sister, Myra Rintamaki, a former ICU nurse at Harborview Hospital in Seattle was particularly helpful in asking the right questions and interpreting the confusing medical terms and abbreviations! My other sister, Trudy Abdo, was there, as was my daughter, Kim Regal, and her husband Mike. My son, Terry O'Malley and wife Jeanie came, as did Steve's three sons and family: Robert, from New York City along with Tom and his wife, Mary and their son, Matthew Tenzin Yarnall; and Steve's son, David and wife, Gail, came down from Washington State. Also arriving was Steve's sister, Nancy Schutte, from Michigan and Steve's brother-in-law, David, from Florida.

We were all united with one goal: "Steve will live"! We held to this conviction through all his ups and downs and even when the advice from some doctors was that the outlook was "hopeless," or that " Steve had under 5% chance of surviving". They underestimated the strengths of Steve and the stubbornness he shares with those of us related to him one way or another. With our Love and Prayers added to by many hundred others, singly and in groups around the world, Steve was certain to win!

Hospital Events

Steve has no conscious memory of his initial accident or of the series of critical events that followed. Each crisis was felt by all of us who followed his clinical ups and downs over his 92-day hospitalization. The procedures to keep Steve alive included:

- ❖ Tracheotomy and assisted ventilation with oxygen
- ❖ Medically-induced coma & paralysis (so that he wouldn't interfere with mechanical ventilation.)
- ❖ Burr hole in head (to release fluid)
- ❖ Central venous lines
- ❖ Medications to maintain blood pressure
- ❖ 7 blood transfusions
- ❖ Rotating bed (Pronation bed – 1st time used at Washoe)
- ❖ Dialysis
- ❖ Exploratory laparotomy
- ❖ PEG feeding tube into duodenum
- ❖ Vena cava filter to prevent blood clots from going to lungs

Email Updates

Hundreds of friends and family anxiously followed Steve via the regular email messages we sent out. Countless others called on the phone to listen to our periodic recorded medical updates on a telephone provided by the Medical Center. These messages provide a moving memory of crisis survival - from the family's perspective. What follows, in *italics* are excerpts from email records. You'll see why we call Steve the "Miracle Man".

The first email sent by our family is from Steve's brother-in-law, David Schutte, to his children. It covers observations through 8 p.m. on January 29.

DAY 2 – January 29, 2000

...Steve has two major threats as of Saturday (Day 2):
1-Pulmonary - He is relying completely on a respirator...and many drips running (Insulin and probably 20 or more drugs); and 2- Cardiovascular - The nurses and physicians are clear about the seriousness of these two threats and say that every 12

hours is critical. Stability may not be achieved for 4-7 days. Family members are on a terribly delicate balance of self-control and mutual support. All are interrupted occasionally by temporary loss of emotional control. The atmosphere is supportive but very difficult...Rather than flowers; please send cards and photos, which are being posted on walls as a large collage.

The collage of photos and cards is of special interest to the nurses and physicians and serves to personalize care for this intubated, multi-tubed, infused, wired-up, comatose, swollen and paralyzed monster - who happens to be my husband. Steve's story continues and although there is stress - of course! - the family keeps a common focus, praying for a healthy survival of this "monster man" - to become a "miracle man."

DAY 3 - Sunday, January 30, 2000
There is no email on Sundays at the Washoe Medical Center but there is a family voice-mail system. Telephone messages are recorded twice daily to report Steve's condition to anyone who calls. Both the email and phone- recorded message services are very useful and appreciated by countless concerned friends and by various prayer groups around the world. In return, I am confident that the force of their love and prayers plays a major role in our goal for Steve's recovery. But at this point in the story there are many tough days ahead of us.

Day 4 -Monday, January 31, 2000
This was nearly the last day of my husband's life. We now know that he has the killer disease called ARDS. The family's response is summed up in my email, which I try to keep as positive as possible:

Steve is still in critical condition. Our hopeful, cautious optimism is faced with the reality that he is the sickest patient in the Intensive Care Unit (ICU)....still requiring medically induced coma and paralysis so that he will not fight the needed assistance with breathing on the ventilator. His inhaled oxygen is down from 100% to

85%, an improvement although ideally he should be around 30%.

Blood pressure is a concern: They need drugs to keep it high enough. They don't know why he can't keep the pressure up by himself. His fragile state keeps them from running all the tests they would like to run.

For now, we need to be realistic and optimistic- realistic in that he is very ill and in critical condition...optimistic in that his numbers are slowly but consistently improving. Keep the focus on today and immediate concerns.

Day 6 - HAPPY BIRTHDAY !

Today - February 2 - is Steve's 66th Birthday and we celebrated with our family, ICU friends and medical staff. We sang "Happy Birthday" to him. Even though still in a coma, Steve showed a response by wrinkling his forehead and actually shedding a tear! We all had happy tears, as we were aware that he seemed to know we were all there for him.

Steve is still critically ill and has many more hurdles to jump, but we have faith he will recover with time. Please continue to keep him in your thoughts and prayers. We truly believe it has helped.

Day 7 - Improving

50% oxygen and 15 PEEP is certainly improved from 6 days ago...and he hasn't required any blood pressure support for two days now. His neurologist has ordered an MRI to help evaluate why his responses are minimal and he is not awakening.

Day 8 - Email Excerpts

...some response to our commands to move his hands and feet...will have another MRI and a brainstem test...has serious sinus infection, being treated with antibiotics...please continue to pray for his recovery.

Day 11 - After the Weekend

...steady progress...semi-conscious...blood pressure down to 70/40 responding to blood transfusions...back to 131/74...had Burr hole drilled in head to drain fluids...CT of chest and abdomen show continued internal bleeding...This morning, despite his critical condition, they propped him up in a special chair to help his circulation--To see him upright was a miracle in itself!

Day 12 – Music and Tubes

...placed in a special chair with a Beethoven classic music video played for stimulation...still on the respirator, his lungs remain a concern to the doctors...his breathing tube is replaced by a tracheotomy and his eating tube...this should make Steve more comfortable...Today Steve mouthed the words "I love you" to me: Do we need to say more?

Day 13 - Lots of Clots

...an ultrasound study shows clots in his right leg so heparin is started and physical therapy stopped to the legs...he is improving neurologically...he puckered a kiss for me and smiled at one of the nurses...we continue to marvel at all the support we are receiving from all of you!

Day 15 - More Clots

Blood clots found in right arm and shoulder as well as right leg...long periods of wakefulness - no longer considered comatose...admits being depressed.

Day 18 - Still Critical

Not much change on the weekend...Steve is still critical, requiring oxygen up to 70% with PEEP of 12...agitated when not on medication...doctors decide not to operate to remove "gunk" from right chest: risks outweigh benefits.

Day 19 - Roto Bed

Steve is sedated and strapped into a Roto-Bed that rolls side-to-side to help circulation and drainage of the lungs.

Day 20 – New Approaches

X-rays today show more clouding...PEEP up to 16 with 60% oxygen. In addition to sedative and paralytic medicine (so that he can't fight the Roto-bed and ventilator), he is being given high doses of corticosteroids (cortisone-like meds) and is being under-ventilated to allow his CO-2 to go way up. These new approaches are supported largely by anecdotal evidence and may carry some long-term side effects. Love and prayers are needed more now than ever...

Day 21 – Outside Informal Consults

The doctors have been very willing to listen and accept suggestions from Steve's friends who are in the medical profession, but not involved with Washoe. The doctors are very open with us, his family, in saying they don't have all the answers. ARDS is one tough illness. Special thanks go to Dr.'s Marv Wayne, Robert Wilson, Phil Dellinger, John Shea, David Cawthon, and Len Hudson who provided suggestions based on their expertise.

Day 22 - 15% Chance of Recovery

This email is written by my sister, Myra Rintamaki, showing her background as an ICU nurse:

> *It's been 3 weeks since Steve's accident and it's been a roller coaster ride since then. Yesterday Steve's condition deteriorated. His kidneys began to fail requiring dialysis. His liver has also begun to fail. Dr. Watson feels Steve's sinus infection may be the primary instigator for his recent deterioration. He has called in an ENT specialist to do a brief procedure to drain the sinuses.*
>
> *Pulmonary wise, the doctors are trying a variety of investigative measures such as high dose steroid therapy, manipulating his CO-2 and pH, pronating him, etc.*
>
> *Percentage wise, Dr. Watson gave Steve a 15% possibility for recovery. He still holds hope and wants to continue full resuscitation measures.*

Day 23 - 13 Family Members

There are 13 family members here to support Steve's recovery. They continue to talk to him lovingly and supportively.

Day 26 - Hanging in There

Hi there to all you Steve Yarnall fans. The fat lady's still singing and Steve's still hanging in there, making progress at a snail's pace, but progress is progress. We continue to orient him and read to him, as well as play soothing music for him.

Day 32 – Bob Yarnall's Comments

Steve is doing better each day. He is still in critical condition in the ICU, but we are back to a state of "cautious optimism." Yesterday, they did an exploratory operation in his abdomen and put in a PEG feeding tube.

His responses are minimal, but he does open his eyes from time to time, and Lynn says that he appeared to move his eyes toward her this morning. Even better, when she asked him to stick his tongue out to show he could understand her, he obliged.

Day 34 – March 1, 2000 - Good News / Bad News

The talk of moving Steve to the ICU at Harborview Hospital in Seattle is still in the works. No date has been set yet, but I was told it could even be as soon as Friday. But as I've learned in the medical field, nothing can be counted on until it actually happens.

Today was sort of a good news/bad news day. The good news is they finally did the EMG. The bad news is they found Steve to have "Critical Care Neuropathy." What this means is that the paralysis of his arms and legs is because the nerves are damaged by his critical illness. The nerves can heal and repair themselves with time.

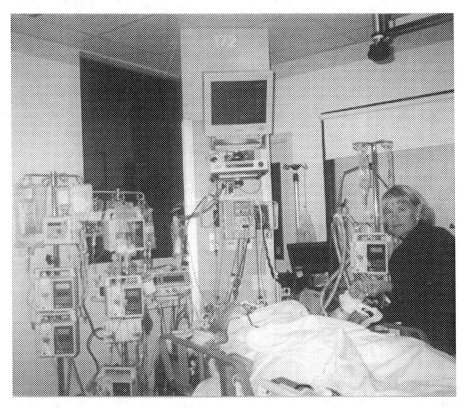

ICU with multiple wires, monitors, infusion equipment, and breathing tube. Lynn stands at bedside.

Can anyone find the patient?

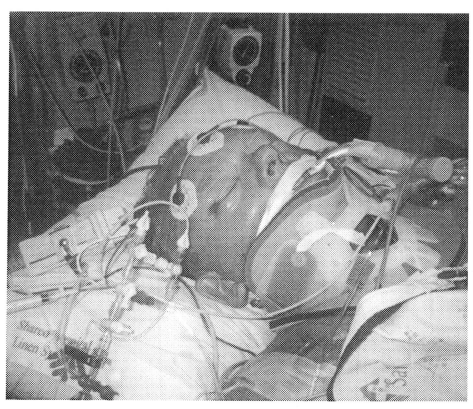

Here's the patient! Notice plastic neck collar, breathing tube through mouth, monitor electrodes on scalp, intravenous site bandaged above right collarbone, and multiple wires and tubes illustrating complexity of modern ICU care.

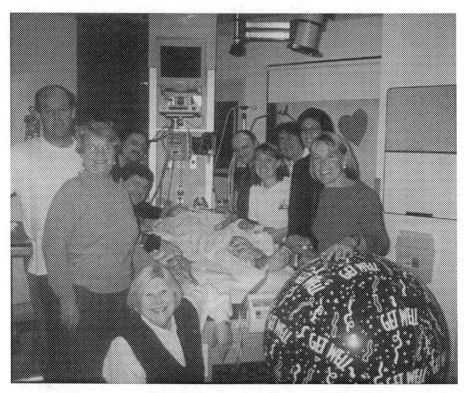

Family members celebrate Steve's 66th Birthday!

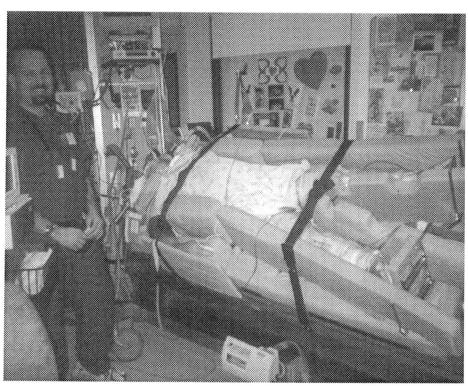

Roto-bed helps balance ventilation and circulation in all areas of the lungs.

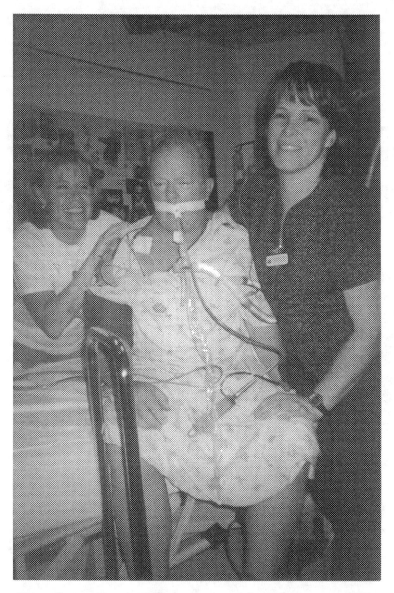

Steve's nurse - Karen W. and wife Lynn help Steve sit on side of bed.

RETURNING HOME TO SEATTLE – Days 35 to 55

This dramatic story of my ARDS continues in Seattle. Although I was conscious, my memory from the following days is very sparse. Therefore, the email records from my wife, Lynn, continue to provide a sense of suspense as this real-life story unfolds.

Day 35 – March 2, 2000

Today was a very special day. When I arrived this morning to visit Steve, I was informed that he was going to be transferred to Harborview within four hours. What a surprise that was to me. Needless to say I was very nervous, but excited.

We arrived at Boeing Field in Seattle on a care-flight Leer jet at 4:15pm with two ICU nurses, two pilots, and myself. The flight took one hour and 20 minutes. From there we were transported in a medic's vehicle to Harborview. Upon arrival, a nurse that used to work for Steve took care of him and made our arrival more comfortable.

Day 37

I finally got to go home for the night. I had over 300 emails on our home computer, which I could not possibly answer.

Days 38-40 – Harborview Trauma ICU

After treatment of a number of problems, Steve was considered one of the more stable trauma ICU patients and moved to Respiratory ICU. We were delighted when he moved his left arm a little. After lying still for so long, any movement brings joy to my heart.

Day 42

They took Steve off the ventilator for about 15 minutes to see how well he could breathe on his own and he did very well without pressure support. He was much more alert today and had a big grin and rolled his eyes when I joked about getting him off the vent and in a wheelchair to do wheelies with him.

Day 44

We need a way to communicate better since we're not good at lip reading and Steve talks too fast and mumbles. We threaten to put lipstick on him so we can read his lips better.

Steve had an incident of bradycardia with a rate of 24 at 6:45am today. His heart rate went back up when the nurse stimulated him by pounding on his chest.

Day 45

Steve had three episodes yesterday when he had a 20-30 second apnea (not breathing) period followed by a low heart rate and decreased consciousness. He quickly regained alertness after these episodes.

Day 47 – March 15, 2000

Steve's body is reacting to seven weeks of bed rest and his muscles and nerves are coming alive again. This is good news, but produces a fair amount of discomfort for Steve with muscle spasms, joint and muscle aches, and an itching sensation. His request is for continuous massage of his extremities and light scratching of his skin.

Day 48

Parking at Harborview is a pain. Most of the family has gotten a parking citation or two. They have a special meter maid just to circle around the hospital, like a pigeon dropping something undesirable.

For any Seafair Clowns who want to stop by after the St. Paddy's Day parade, beware of Nurse Cratchet who limits visitors to two at a time – but for you guys we have special permission.

Day 49 – Graduation Day from ICU to Neurology Floor

It's Friday night and Steve has to move to the Neurology floor to make room in the ICU for the St. Paddy's Day celebrators. Steve had a great surprise today when a wagonload of Seafair Clowns stopped by. Steve managed to con a few of them into scratching his arms.

In spite of the parking crisis, the clowns pulled the clown vehicle onto the sidewalk in front of the hospital and came right in.

Day 50

Though Steve was still too weak to turn himself over in bed, he spoke today when his trach was plugged. He maintains his sense of humor in singing his first words – "la, la, la."

Day 52

Steve had a wonderful day today. The respiratory therapist came in and buttoned Steve's trach opening so he can talk. The good news is he can communicate with us; the bad news is he hasn't stopped talking, singing, and joking. I guess he has eight weeks to catch up on, and he's doing it in the first couple of hours. What a sense of relief it is for Steve to be able to communicate.

Day 55

Today's big milestone…Steve stood up, though helped by therapists. Everything exhausts him immensely. He told me today that lifting a matchbox was like lifting 100 pounds.

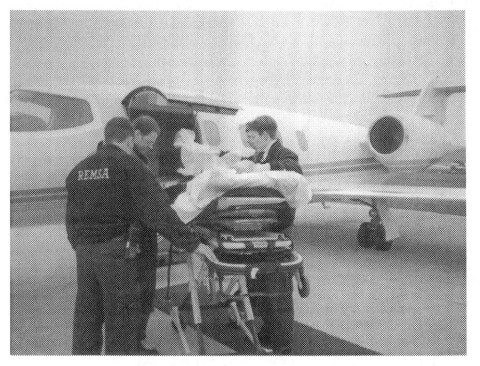

**Getting ready to load Steve on
jet to go from Reno to Seattle.**

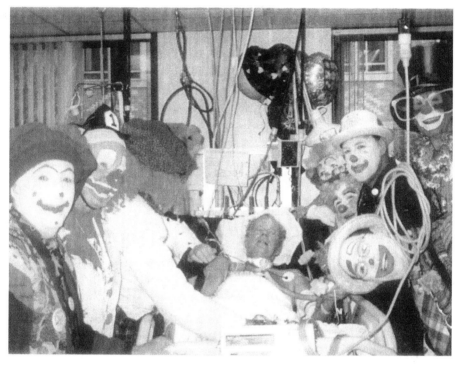

Visiting Seafair Clowns in Harborview ICU... "a first" for ICU care... elicits a faint clown smile from Steve, who himself has been a Seafair Clown for 24 years.

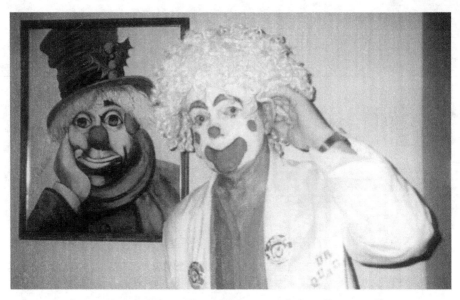

The author, Dr. Yarnall, as his Seafair Clown character, "Dr. Quack" in 2002, two years after his hospitalization for ARDS

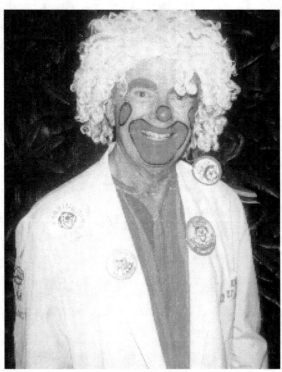

REHABILITATION
"NO PAIN - NO GAIN"
Days 56 to 92

I remember these days struggling to get back some capability to do normal activities of daily living. I was grateful to my family and friends for all their love and prayers and personal attention. They continued to inform the network of email followers regarding my progress.

Day 56– March 23, 2000
Myra Rintamaki writes, after Steve's transfer to the Rehab floor:

Steve remains short of breath and seems to think (as a cardiologist would) that it is related to his heart (cardiomyopathy). He still has to be fed because his arm strength and coordination aren't there yet.

Day 57
It is amazing how far Steve has come in the past month. He is already thinking of a title for the book he's going to write.

They're having a Kingdome implosion party complete with a funky harps and flute kind of band at 7 a.m. Sunday on the balcony off the unit. We are thinking of selling tickets for the birdseye view of the implosion.

Steve's grandson, Matthew Tensin, and his great niece, Jaylinn were there to visit him today. They are both two years old and very entertaining but I'm sure Steve was glad they got to go home for dinner.

Day 60
Steve had another "first" today. He held a glass by himself and took a drink of water. It makes me so grateful for what I have when I watch Steve work through these basic but important steps. It is a reminder to us all not to take things for granted.

Steve has a "memory book" to record questions for the staff that they can answer in writing.

Day 61 – March 28, 2000 – Myra (Lynn's sister)

Steve is sleeping like a baby, waking up only when the nurse comes in to give him medicine – you know the drill – wake the patient up to give him a sleeping pill. Steve got his trach tube out at last and is doing well on two liters of oxygen. He went to the hospital gym and laid on the mat to practice lifting himself on his elbow – powerful stuff for the "miracle man". His will to move is stronger than his physical body is able to accomplish.

Steve has lost 25 pounds in the last 61 days. I offered to give him a fat graft.

Day 62 - First Message dictated by Steve Yarnall

For my next trick, I think I'll have a seizure, fall 30 feet from a chairlift, be airlifted to Washoe Medical Center in Reno and almost die, be intubated, get ARDS, have a feeding tube and after 35 days in the ICU, get transported to Seattle for continued care in Harborview ICU and Rehab center…come to think about it, I've already done that so I'll have to think of something else to top that act.

This whole experience has taught me the importance of supportive friends, loving family members, prayer, positive thinking, humor, and skilled physicians with first class facilities. A family member has stayed with me each night since the accident to fill in the inevitable gaps in nursing care, such as "I'm thirsty" or "I have to go pee pee". Having a tracheotomy for over a month is not easy for someone who likes to talk, although Lynn didn't get any back-talk during that period. I'm particularly appreciative of the time and effort put forth by my wife, Lynn in handling our personal and professional affairs. (Will she ever get caught up on sleep loss?)

I sincerely appreciate the many cards, flowers, balloons and messages received everyday for the past 62 days. My room looks like a florist and balloon shop. We're sorry we can't thank everyone individually for their thoughtfulness, but there are just sooo many.

Now that my prognosis is better than death, I'm struggling primarily with painful, tingling, weak hands and legs. My exact plans are uncertain, but I would like to return to a limited practice and more writing and speaking.

We're planning one or more "new arrivals" in May – from our Golden Retriever, Cinco de Mayo, not Lynn. Helping to care for the new puppies should be a therapeutic part of my recovery. Woof woof!

Again, I appreciate your love and caring.

Have a Happy Heart,

Steve

Day 63 - March 30, 2000 - Steve's Second Message

Some people may have thought I was full of ____, but after the suppository, I'm at least 3 days less. In addition to my explosion and the implosion of the Kingdome, other things have been exploding in a big way too. Another high point was standing today unassisted for 3 seconds. I was able to feed myself a little bit but still needed assistance for most of the meal (almost as good as a 2-year old). As of today, I can hold a glass by myself. But, it's hard to get a good gin and tonic here.

I had my first shower in 63 days today, sitting in a wheelchair. It sure felt great! Ross, the speech therapist, and I are challenging each other with riddles and puzzles. For example, Charlotte's mother had 3 children: The first 2 were named Penny and Nickel. What was the name of the third? Answer in tomorrow's email.

Day 66 - April 2, 2000 - Steve

I missed April Fool's Day because we were all fooled by the weather – it was sunny.

I continue to make slow but steady progress. My major disability remains the weakness, stiffness, and tingling in my fingers which makes it impossible to do common tasks such as eating, writing, and turning the pages of a book.

By the way, the answer to the riddle in the last message is as Linda Stern said concisely in her reply, "Charlotte, of course!"

Day 68 - April 4, 2000 - Steve

Today I had a visit from a very special friend and artist, Jeff Nicholson. Jeff is a C4 Quad who draws remarkable illustrations by holding a pencil in his mouth. He is currently working on a beautiful color picture of a scene with an eagle in it. Jeff and I shared issues about living without the use of one's hands. Jeff's positive attitude inspired me. It's amazing what one can do in spite of physical limitations. Jeff's mother, LeeAnna, has worked as my medical stenographer for over ten years. She acts as Jeff's agent and would be happy to send you information on how to buy one of Jeff's prints.

Day 77 - April 13, 2000 – Lynn

These last few days are the end of an era. Steve's medical practice will be closed as of Saturday, April 15, 2000. It is sad, but in a way, it is also good. Change is good, even if it is with a bit of hard luck. Steve will always find other ways to challenge himself. He's already thinking of a million ways. Thanks to his office staff who have been so helpful in organizing this closure.

Day 82 - April 18, 2000 – Lynn

Steve came home tethered to a 50-foot oxygen line that followed him around delivering 2 liters of oxygen. Steve will come home for an overnight pass this Saturday and Sunday in preparation for his discharge on April 28th. We are having an Easter brunch at our house on Sunday. What a celebration of life. Can you imagine? We feel so grateful to have Steve home to celebrate.

Day 88 - April 24, 2000 – Myra

Easter Sunday was great! Steve's son, Bob, flew in from New York and Steve's sister, Nancy, flew in from Michigan. Steve's progress is truly remarkable. Was the experience in Reno just a bad dream? Lynn still hasn't had the opportunity to slow down after Steve's accident. She has a lot of "SISU" – that's Finnish for determination and stubbornness. It gets her through her ultra-distance runs and has gotten her though this one great marathon.

My family joins me in thanking all of you for your great support throughout this ordeal. We thank those of you who prayed for Steve and the rest of us. We thank all of the medical people who are out there that were responsible for Steve's medical needs and remember, miracles can happen no matter how strong the odds are against you. I remember being in the waiting room at Washoe hospital after Steve took a turn for the worse. Dr. Watson said, " Steve has a 15% chance of survival, but there is nothing that's happened that's irreversible, so let's not let Mother Nature have him without a fight."

Thank you Dr. Bob Watson for being a fighter, for staying in the ring with us, giving us hope, and encouraging all the other staff at Washoe. Thanks to all the staff who shared in Steve's survival. Thanks to everyone who prayed for Steve and sent cards expressing their love for him. It so unbelievable that Steve is coming home on Friday. A special thanks goes to Lynn who has been by Steve's side throughout this event.

HOME CARE

Lynn and I hired a Home Healthcare provider, Janine Koch, to help me while Lynn was at work. Janine kept a daily log, which jogs my memory of how dependent I was at that time. It also reminds me of how much I appreciated a massage of my tight muscles. The following three email messages conclude the story of my 92-day hospital stay and the next six days at home.

Day 92 - April 28, 2000 – DISCHARGE DAY!!
Nancy Schutte (Steve's sister)

From chairlift to toboggan to helicopter to hospital to ambulance to Leer jet to ambulance to hospital to wheelchair to walker. Day 92 and Steve Yarnall is home. Do you hear that, Dr. Robert Watson and the Washoe staff? Steve Yarnall is home. Be proud! I watched him slowly walk through the front door with a huge smile on his face. He uses a walker for the short trips and a wheelchair for the long hauls – in time he will dance. He uses special hand utensils for eating – in time he will carve the turkey. He moves slowly – in time he will chase Cinco's puppies. He speaks quickly and mumbles slightly – but with concentration his words are loud and clear and his wonderful tenor singing voice is better than ever.

After weeks of silence, he now laughs at his own jokes. He shows excitement and pleasure at each card, note, gift, call, or visit. He has started looking at pictures from Reno and quietly cries at the magnitude of all that has happened. Thankfully he remembers nothing. We tell him everyday about all of you – your vigil, prayers, and love kept us strong so we could be strong for Steve. Each of us found our individual faith strengthened, witnessing the power of prayer and excellent medical treatment.

And through it all, there has been Lynn. She slept on couches, floors, chairs, and hospital beds. She is my hero, and a huge ingredient in my brother's recovery. Remember, people with ARDS as critical as Steve's usually don't survive.

Another thank you to Myra, Lynn's sister, who I call Mapes and Steve calls his "wife-in-law". Her medical training, gentleness, and persistence to have the very best care for Steve reassured us.

Our family became closer as we drew together as a team. From seven states we kept in constant touch. We became more respectful of life and we learned the true meaning of friendships…all of you.

April 30, 2000 – At Home - Day 2 - Lynn

"Oh what a beautiful morning. Oh what a beautiful day. I've got a wonderful feeling…"

It's been a long time since I've felt like singing…today I feel like singing forever.

What a blessing to be able to sleep together in our own bed. It's fun to be back home with our dog, Cinco. It's great to be able to just step outside the door and feel the fresh air and sunshine, instead of stale hospital air. And it's just wonderful to be back home, PERIOD!

I am so grateful for the good things in life, which include all our family and friends. Steve and I will both be forever grateful to everyone for everything they have done for us. I am especially appreciative for the caring, thoughtful cards, phone call, flowers, gifts, and prayers that were sent to me as well as to Steve. I'm thankful to my employer WPAS, and to my department manager Cherri Jennings for allowing me to take the necessary time off. I also want to thank my co-workers for covering my duties while I was away.

June 4, 2000 – At Home - Day 6 - Lynn

Steve requires a caretaker to help with morning physical needs such as showering, dressing, eating, and taking meds. He also goes to Northwest Hospital Rehab Center 3 days a week. Steve still has limited use of his fingers, which are still numb and tingling. Other than this, Steve's general strength is improving. He is off supplemental oxygen, but he still gets out of breath very easily. He even mowed the lawn the other day. He was exhausted, but had a feeling of accomplishment.

He is planning to resume a part-time medical practice in two months. He is very anxious to get back to medicine. He loves helping others even though he's the one who needs help right now. He feels he still has what it takes to be a very good doctor.

It's Steve's idea to have a "Celebration of Life" party to take the place of what would have been a funeral. We will have a Dixieland Jazz Band, the "Ain't no Heaven Seven". This is a group of doctors led by Terry Rogers and including Steve's long-time friend Ward Kennedy on trombone, and others.

Conclusion – June 15, 2002 -
Steve -4 1/2 months after accident

In concluding this chapter, I want to say how much I appreciate the way Lynn and family members kept everyone informed about my progress with ARDS. These email messages were forwarded to many other individuals across the country. I am amazed that I continue to meet people who say, "Oh, you're the guy who fell off the chairlift!" Reading copies of these email records two years later gives me the sense that I'm reading about someone other than myself. The written messages document the intensity of love and prayer, which were "Beyond Medicine", and important elements of my healing. Although I continue to have some residual disabilities from ARDS, I am grateful for all I am able to do, which includes returning to active medical practice – and writing this book.

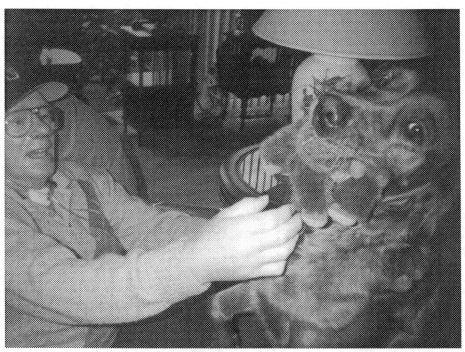

**Steve, with happy tears, is presented
a welcoming home gift by Cinco.**

Christmas Reflections 2000
by Robert Yarnall

From the first phone call I received in January to the wonderful Celebration of Life in July, the past year has offered a hands-on lesson in miracles. At Christmas we celebrate life. And here are my thoughts on the whole thing, as it happened, taken directly from my journal. In the movies miracles happen all at once, and rather easily. But here are the details, the downs and ups, of actually living through one.

Selections from my journal:

Day 7 (2/3/2000)

I have to go on, all of us do, as if Steve's progress will be steady and will lead to a fully interactive person like the one we knew just a few days ago. Today, after yesterday's responsiveness and interaction – squeezing of hands, opening eyes and wiggling toes on command – he is back to zero responsiveness. Yesterday we celebrated his birthday and he seemed to cry when Nancy read her birthday card aloud. Right after she said "M-I-K" (more in kitchen), he convulsed, furrowed his brows and seemed to tear up. Today we got nothing from him....

I find myself imagining delivering a speech, either at his celebration of life, or else a eulogy. He would want us to celebrate life and get together after his full recovery and I want to say, out loud and in front of the whole family, what he means to me. Why get together just at funerals as he so often says. And by extension, why just give a eulogy just at a funeral? We can choose to celebrate life *now*. He has shown me that, not just *said* it. He arranged the cruise and the family reunions. Those are real, not abstract. So I intend to deliver a speech, a living eulogy, at his celebration.

Day 22 (2/18/2000)

I don't even know at this moment if my father is alive. Flying to San Francisco, hoping to connect to Reno, I'm out of touch during what are his most fragile times. There are no promises now, little hope extended. 15% chance, the doctor estimates. We're all coming out as quickly as we can....

Hard to accept any of this as God's will, unless he recovers and inspires others as a result; that seems God-worthy. But I, we, can never know....

I love him and am not ready to let him go. There's so much more we could do and be together. Please.

Day 29 (2/25/2000)

A week of miracles. I arrived late last Friday night to a happy ICU Waiting Room, an immediate visual relief. Lynn said, "You arrived at a good time." He had stabilized and since then has continued to get better....

His rehabilitation will be much longer now, a small price to pay. The prayers and the treatment are working, I believe together. Left brain and right brain support giving Steve life.

Day 32 (2/28/2000)

The events of a life do not edit neatly into a story. Life is about waiting between events and, in fact, maybe it's this between time where life really happens. Trained by TV and film, something in me expects more drama, more events, more easily and quickly defined resolutions. But patience is a virtue and it's just like my dad somehow to teach it to us in this way....

Day 34 (3/1/2000)

It looks like he'll go home this week, maybe on Friday, i.e. 3/3. His rehab will take months; hopefully there is no permanent nerve damage.

I seem to have confidence in his recovery....

Four Months Later (July, 2000)

We'll all gather to celebrate Steve this weekend. So much happened in February and March. It now seems like another life.

Time spent at Washoe was its own distinct reality. Our world so focused, so narrowly focused, that we didn't even see the whole ICU for days, as if it didn't exist. As Steve improved, suddenly the world expanded a bit at a time. They've installed a kitchen in the ICU, and plaques on the wall.

Tense times coming from the airport in a taxi. The driver smells of cigarettes. For him it's another fare, hopes for a tip. Try to stay casual. The last thing I want is to discuss this with a cab driver, to share and open up in a 5-minute drive. No, I needed to prepare, each time, for what I'd see.

The waiting, all that waiting. First in New York City, then on the plane. All alone all that time. Until I stepped out of that cab and went to find the ICU. Heart pounding that first time, all the uncertainties – of how he'd look, what state of crisis would he be in. Being greeted in the ICU Waiting Room, that wonderful little blue room with the flexible furniture, the two phones, the few child-sized chairs, no windows. A community of families together in fear and hope.

And now, arriving, not alone anymore. The news encouraging enough that we play cards, we talk, even all go out to dinner.

And the second time, the uncertainty even stronger. Will he be alive? It's a very relevant question. Coming across the country on President's Day week-end, the flights packed, cancellations due to weather. I make it somehow, have waited to hear any news, the thought of hearing it on a phone, alone in an airport, is unbearable, in case the news is bad. So again to the taxis. I say a prayer. He's in God's hands. I know where to go this time and I move through those corridors imagining what I'll see – grief, happiness, no one there. Each possibility has its meaning.

And then relief, huge relief, as I look in the window to the waiting room. My family is there, chatting casually, relaxed. I know he is alive. I've made it in time. The hope is higher. I arrived at a good time, as Lynn put it. And from then on we remain as hopeful as we can. The prognosis is still around 15%. We look for small signs.

Myra asks the questions. We feed ours to her. She filters and translates. The doctors try to drive home: please don't think that far ahead, let's just try to get through this next day, this next procedure or test. He seems stable. We monitor, some even graph, his progress. His peep, his oxygen concentration, a thousand lights.

The machines change. The cards keep coming in. The voicemail updated daily. The email updated Monday to Friday. We're busy all day, supporting each other, getting and disseminating information, calling family, opening cards.

Then the dinner hour. We're forced to see the outside world.

Not allowed to visit Steve. Lynn always has a pager, ready to be contacted the instant anything changes. She reminds the nurses of this. Our world has expanded from our corner of the waiting room to the town of Reno. We come back from our walks. We play Celebrity. It becomes an obsession. We comment that Steve managed to get another family reunion together. We imagine the reunion t-shirt. Something with a ski lift. The Washoe Newsletter has several pieces of advice for safety, ending with, "Never jump from a ski lift."

We watch the Millionaire show. We, now the old hands, welcome the new families, commiserate. The couple from North Carolina – their son Kale keeps improving. There are people here we would probably never speak to otherwise. Here they become like family. Politics, religion, accents, backgrounds, all of it so irrelevant. It all boils down to this. We're here for love. Hoping, every moment, to keep grief away – though it seems like it's ready to appear at any moment. A test result or sudden crisis. A turn for the worse. That room is all about waiting. It becomes a full time occupation. Filling that waiting.

The cafeteria. Those big cookies at lunch. The espresso cart with their file of Frequent Buyer cards, their sign that says, "Friends don't let friends drink Starbucks." Once or twice, maybe on a week-end when the cart was closed, someone made a Starbuck's run. A huge order of coffee, eight or nine beverages, several thousand dollars.

In New York I kept a lamp burning, an eternal flame next to my dad's Millennium photo, holding the January 1st Seattle Times. The flame goes day and night. I even light a back-up flame with the original flame every morning when I refill the oil. It never goes out. And every day I look at his picture and observe and command, "You keep getting better."

He disobeyed me once. Got the whole family very upset. Steve slipped perilously close to the past tense. Slowly we expanded that tense back out again. But talk about living in a day-tight compartment. It was, in fact, tight - and very much like a claustrophobic compartment.

What I admire about my dad was in evidence at Washoe:
He touches people, he's obviously affected many lives, inspired people. Look at all the support that poured in – cards, emails, voicemails, packages, prayers, letters.

The value of *celebrating* life for now. The reunion. *Doing* it.
Passion for his career.
Adventure
Socializing – again, all the people he's known
Consideration…
Discussion and philosophizing.
A blessing – More Life. The giving of life. Engage life.

Postscript-Four months later - July 2000

I'm happy. I was able to speak at my father's Celebration of Life party…. I spoke of my dad as a blessing. A blessing: more life. Through his career, the people he's touched, his recovery, the way prayer and people and medicine all came together to bless us all. We've all been given more life through this - most obviously Steve, of course. But I know and appreciate life, the people and things in it now, more.

Lynn, you were like a hurricane force at Washoe, tirelessly working to save my father's life and inspiring us all in ways impossible to measure.

And Steve, even though you don't remember hearing us, thank you for listening to our prayers, and coming back to inspire us again.

II SIX ELEMENTS OF HEALING

Clearly there are many " elements of healing" beyond traditional medical care. The reality that these are difficult to study may cause a physician to overlook the importance of these elements. I have chosen six elements which stood out in my experience and memory in recovering from ARDS. In the sections that follow I will discuss my experience with Love, Prayer, Touch, Humor, Music, and Pets.

LOVE – A HEALING FORCE

" Listening is the first duty of love."
-Dale Turner[i]

While I was in a coma I did my duty of love and listened. And what I received was LOVE - love from the bedside presence of my wife and family, love from the physicians, nurses and staff who cared for me; love from friends across the country; and love in the prayers of countless persons the world around.

I put "Love" first in the six elements of healing, which contributed to the miracle of my recovery from the jaws of ARDS. When I awoke after nearly dying in my ventilator-supported coma. I felt an overwhelming feeling of being loved. That love was a deep caring for me with the power of prayer whether from individual at my bedside, across the country or on the other side of the world. My spirit was supported by this love, which, in turn, helped the healing of my mind and body. In the face of what was considered "hopeless" by some of my consulting physicians (but not Dr. Watson), love was a prayer answered by my recovery in spite of the odds.

This love was given to me as a gift, as it was given to Meg, and Carrie, and Sheridan, and Eileen and all those whose stories are included in this book. Therefore I will not be quoting testimonies about "Love" in all these cases. Instead, I will be looking at "Love" itself and how it might work as an element of healing – beyond Medicine. Love is a force, which is stronger than any medicine. Love itself is a medicine and a special, precious gift, which can't be bought. Love is a gift, which the more you give, the more you have.

When I emerged from my coma I was overwhelmed by the 100's of cards expressing support for me with Love and Prayers. It was later, as I started to write this book, that I realized how much in love with love I have been and how much credit goes to many sources for my current feelings about Love.

Every one of the crisis stories sent to me for this book mentioned supportive Love as an element of their care. But, how are we to interpret "Love" as a force for healing? To begin with, let us agree that "Love" is referred to as a central aspect of all major religions and our relation to God. (Later in this book we will see that love is the major component of the man-dog relationship as well.)

Christians and Jews both profess the Bible's Old Testament. The Bible starts with the concept of God as a judgmental, punishing, rule-making, super-Being. Later in time He expresses Himself through Jesus as a God of forgiveness and love. "For God so loved the world that he gave his only begotten son" are words I learned early in Sunday school. And "Love thy neighbor as thyself" carries the double duty to love yourself first and then care for others as yourself. ("Do unto others as you would have others do unto you" is always a challenge but makes a good start in helping me care for (Love?) others.) Here are some paraphrased parts from Chapter 13 of First Corinthians[ii]:

No matter how successful I am, and even if I'm strong enough to move mountains, I am nothing if I don't have Love in my life;
Prophesies will fail; Knowledge will vanish and change; Love never fails;
We ultimately have Faith, Hope and Love - - and the greatest of these is LOVE.

However we define "LOVE," and in whatever religion we choose, "LOVE" is a central concept. It continues to amaze me that no-one copyrighted the one word title, "LOVE", for a book until Leo Buscaglia did it in 1972[iii]. Although Leo passed on in 1998, his message continues through his spirit, his books and an active website: www.buscaglia.com. This site is dedicated to the memory and works of Leo Buscaglia, best-selling author and professor on the experience of love.

In the Buscaglia chat room, under the topic, "Keep love alive" I entered a brief blurb about my ARDS titled, "Love kept me alive." Here is one of the responses:

> *Dr. Yarnall,*
> *I was so glad to hear your statement on your experience and the amazing amount of people that had given you their expressions of love and their prayers for your survival. I honestly feel your excitement only by reading your miracle! I know that when prayers are said results occur by the energy passed by faith one to another. From your words and your sharing such a positive message that shows me one person out of thousands the miraculous results are so moving to read. There are so many in the world who have experienced LOVE in that magnitude that changes a person for the greater purpose of Love being kept alive in our world.*
> *Love is a light that knows all human life as worth everything and more. Love is survival and growth to a far greater magnitude that I have ever realized*
> > *Keith*

My reply to Keith agreed with his model of Love and Prayer as united forces for healing.

Buscaglia's poetic prose is typified in this passage on our opportunity to make our love felt:

> *The majority of us lead quiet, unheralded lives as we pass through this world. There will most likely be no ticker-tape parades for us, no monuments created in our honor. But that does not lessen our possible impact, for there are scores of people waiting for someone just like us to come along; people who will appreciate our compassion, our encouragement, who will need our unique talents. Someone who will live a happier life merely because we took the time to share what we had to give. Too often we underestimate the power of a touch, a smile, a kind word, a listening ear, an honest*

compliment, or the smallest act of caring, all of which have the potential to turn a life around. It's overwhelming to consider the continuous opportunities there are to make our love felt.

Leo Buscaglia—*"Born for Love"*

There are many perceived <u>outcomes</u> of "love" from the effect on an individual to groups and nations for world peace:

The fruit of love is service.
The fruit of service is peace.
And peace begins with a smile.
-Mother Teresa

It is no accident that Mother Teresa wrote the forward to Dr. Lester Sauvage's book "The Open Heart". Dr. Sauvage[iv] and his patients present a series of inspiring stories, which he says brought him closer to God, as he believes they will also do for the reader. Mother Teresa's opening quote is:

God has created each one of us for greater things –
To love and to be loved.
Let us give each other not only our hands to serve,
but also our hearts to love with kindness and humility.

Dr. Sauvage gave both his hands and his heart to his patients for 33 years and founded the world-renowned Hope Heart Institute in 1959 as a center for research and education. The Institute continues to be a world leader in these functions.

An old quote passed on by the Quakers is: *"Work is Love made visible."* This is wonderful for those of us who are "workaholics" but has meaning to everyone. But how does work, smiling, making our love felt, etc. have an impact on a critically ill patient, such as one with ARDS?

I believe that "Love," in the sense we are using the word, works through the very same force as Prayer. Granted, as discussed in the section on Prayer, we have less understanding of how prayer works than we have of how gravity works – but that shouldn't lessen our belief in prayer. Just because gravity, prayer and love are invisible forces, we should not doubt their reality.

The insight from my experience is that the expressions of Love for me were the same as prayers, and that Prayers for me were the same as love. Further, I have come to believe in Prayer and Love as actual forces, as "Elements of Healing – Beyond Medicine". It can be said that this belief is based on "Faith" – in a demeaning sense, in contrast to "Science." I accept the label of "Faith" in the sense of reasonable belief based on open-minded observations in many cases. All "Science" begins this way, with deeper understanding at a later date. Or am I still to believe the world is flat?

"Evidence-based" Medicine must not be fearful of looking at new evidence, even if it fails to fit into existing models. Love is a force that can be used along with the always – changing therapies of current medical care. Physicians, nurses and all those in contact with patients have the opportunity and choice to use Love and Prayer in patient care. And I have heard stories where the attitude of food servers and room cleaners made the difference in patients who were about to give it up.

Not everyone will be as fortunate as I (and others) to have spouses, family members, friends and medical care providers at every level caring for them with such Love. That gives more opportunity for each of us to be "Love-Therapists"(LTs) in the context of healing. For those who want to have a greater understanding of Love as a healing force, there are several books I would suggest.

Love, Medicine & Miracles[v]

Dr. Bernie Siegel is famous for his book "Love, Medicine & Miracles" dealing with lessons he has learned about self-healing from his experience with "exceptional patients". Bernie notes, "It isn't easy to put love under a microscope". He states he is trying to help people here and now on an individual basis, "letting others take care of the statistics".

Bernie is a believer in the power of love and states,

> *"I am convinced that unconditional love is the most powerful stimulant of the immune system. If I told patients to raise their blood levels of immune globulins or killer T cells, no one would*

*know how. But if I can teach them to love themselves and others fully, the same changes happen automatically. The truth is: **love heals**."*

The journal <u>Lancet</u> Vol.357, Pg.757 reports doctors who show warmth and reassurance with patients have better outcomes than emotionally cooler colleagues. The relaxation of the more warmly treated patients is associated with improved immune function (Source: Hope Health Letter – www.HopeHealth.com/hhl).

Love is classically related to seeking the love of God, as a two-way street, not just seeking love and favors from God, but expressing our love of God through our love of others. Love, expressed to the critically ill patient, is a type of prayer for that individual.

As the Quakers say, "there is that of God in every man", so expressing love for another person is also expressing love for God.

Siegel says,

"Choose to love and make others happy, and your life will change because you will find happiness and love in the process. The first step towards inner peace is to decide to give love, not receive it."

These ideas of Siegel relate to the rehabilitative phase of ARDS and similar critical illnesses when it is easy to feel sorry for ones self. I recall one of my first thoughts after regaining consciousness was, "Oh boy … now I have something to write a book about!" I am grateful to God for having the mind and strength to fulfill this opportunity with the help of my family and friends. Part of my strength came from my earlier studies, including a book by Gerald Jampolsky, M.D., *"Love Is Letting Go of Fear*[vi]*"*. The basic precept of his book is revealed in the title: one cannot feel fear and love at the same time. Therefore, nurturing our ability to love is freeing us from the burden of fear.

Leo Buscaglia in his book, *"Living, Loving and Learning"* starts out by discussing love as a behavior modifier: *"Every time you learn something you become something new"*. The most important thing for a loving person to learn is to love and value himself. I always visualize this in terms of the advice given on airlines about putting on your own oxygen mask first if you are traveling with someone who might need help.

The really important learning in life comes <u>from</u> life, not from school. We are shaped by the love of others and by the love we give to others. God speaks to us through rainbows, that wonder of nature which requires both sunshine and rain. Just because we can't catch a rainbow doesn't make it unreal. Life and Death may be seen as ends of a rainbow and Death may not be the ending, but rather the beginning of another adventure.

Death is a great reminder of the importance of living each day to the fullest with lots of love and laughter. There is a connection between love and laughter which we will explore in the section on Humor.

SUMMARY

Love is a healing force for critically ill patients as it was in my case with ARDS. The "Love-force" was like a "Prayer-force" from the many people who felt love and the intense desire for my survival. It pleases me to know that those who felt love for me also received the healing power of Love for themselves.

---

[i] Dale Turner – Grateful Living, High Tide Press 1998, 283pp,
> *Similar to his first collection of SeattleTimes columns in book form "Different Seasons".*
> *This book is a delightful, stimulating collection of essays on grateful living, taking life with*
> *"gratitude instead of for granted" (Chesterton)*

[ii] The Bible, New Testament, Corinthians I, Chapter 13, verses 1-13
> *Probably the most quoted chapter on Love in world literature, starting with the words,* "Although I speak with the tongues of angels but have not love, I have become sounding brass or a clanging cymbal."

[iii] Leo Buscaglia, Love, Fawcett Crest, New York, 1972, 207 pp (paperback)
> " Living, Loving & Learning, Fawcett Columbine, New York, 1982, 264 pp
> " (other books: Born To Love; Personhood); ...
> *Buscaglia, without doubt, is the best known author on the topic of "Love"*

in American   literature, Even after his death his spirit lives on through his web site: www.buscaglia.com.

[iv] Lester R. Sauvage, M.D., The Open Heart, Health Communications, Inc., 1996, 248pp, paperback

This is a series of patient stories of "Hope, Healing and Happiness", starting with a forward by Mother Teresa and a former U.S. Surgeon General, C.E.Koop. Sauvage's love for each patient is legendary, and their love for him is apparent in their stories as they tell them.

Bernie Siegel, "Love, Medicine & Miracles", Harper & Row Publishers, New York, 1986, 244pp hardback.

The classic work on self healing of "exceptional cancer patients", followed by many more publications, videos and public appearances.

[v] Gerald Jampolsky, Love Is Letting Go of Fear, Bantam Books, 1970, 131pp, paperback.

Jampolsky gives credit to "A Course in Miracles" as a basis for this national best seller. The concepts of the 12 lessons in this book are as vital today as they were over 30 years ago.

PRAYER -
A PROVEN ELEMENT
FOR HEALTH AND HEALING

*"More things are wrought by prayer
than this world dreams of"*
Lord Alfred Tennyson (1869)

One of my first memories upon waking from my "medical coma" (induced to allow mechanical ventilation without my resistance) was reading the many cards sent to me. First, the number - which was over 500, astounded me. Second, I immediately felt the message of Love and Prayer for me. I was truly struck by the number and the similarity of the messages. I felt uplifted by the Love and strengthened by the Prayer-force for me. Because of this, I have come to a new concept of Prayer and its power.

Previously, I believed in the power of prayer for myself or for you IF you knew about it. Although I had prayed for others and for general goals such as "world peace," I was not certain this could produce results. Possibly, I thought, if the person I prayed for was aware of my prayer, there could be some benefit. I changed my beliefs as a result of the miracle of my recovery from near-death with ARDS. I was moved by the evidence of all the cards and calls referring to Prayer. I later learned that, in addition to the individual prayers, there had been numerous prayer groups praying for my recovery. I was told of various Christian congregations, Quaker Meetings, Jewish Synagogues, Buddhist Groups and others, including many non-church groups, all around the world who had prayed for my recovery. I am convinced that prayer played an important role in my healing. This healing effect did not depend on distance, my awareness, or the particular religious denomination or sect of those praying for me.

Though I can not fully understand God, or how prayer works, this does not block my belief based on personal experience, and reinforced by the convictions and stories of many others from all walks of life over many eras of human existence. "We live by the stories we tell", said Walter Bowman at a summer "retreat" which I attended at Holden Village over 10 years ago.[i] Walter Bowman said we have a choice of which story to live by, and that he had chosen the Christian story. But, he noted, he respected other stories and those who live by them. This "Story Theology" attracted me because it was open-minded while still allowing convictions to live by. And one of my convictions - stories I live by - is that the prayers for my recovery from ARDS were an important element of my healing.

Trust in prayer alone may be harmful to your health! God works through humans to bring help to those in need. As a physician I have had patients and families refuse needed surgery, coronary care, or other care based solely on trust in prayer. I advise my patients to accept God's help through the hands of healers which help us meet achievable goals.

Prayer is closely related to Goals. Praying for a good outcome, as well as visualizing how it will be, is important elements of healing. As I was recovering from my ARDS, I visualized and prayed for my return to an active medical practice and for completing this book. While accepting my losses and limitations, I have accomplished these goals - with the help of God and many loving individuals.

In his book, "Man's Search for Meaning", Victor Frankl discusses "Logotherapy". Logotherapy seeks to help an individual find meaning in life and personal goals. This remains one of the most important parts of my medical philosophy and practice, as I help patients find, "What do you want to live for and do?" I recall an aphorism which says, "If you don't know where you're going, you're probably going nowhere!" And this, in turn, reminds me of Joel Goodman's well-posed puzzle:

What do you read when you see:

"OPPORTUNITYISNOWHERE"?

Most people read this as saying "opportunity is nowhere". A few jokers read this as "opportunity - I snow here!" But we are challenged to move from the first interpretation to another, imbedded in the same message: "Opportunity is Now Here"! I choose to believe that "Opportunity IS Now Here" for you and for me, even if it's hard to find. This may be the place for the prayer, "God, please show me the way!" And the answer may show us "….unity is now here" - - and ignore the "op port"! Indeed, unity is part of opportunity. Just as "Chance favors the prepared mind", so does unity of prayer favor the opportunity of results from those prayers, as I visualize the power of prayer, for whatever outcome…

Many happy outcomes may be prayed for in medical crises, but I believe the central prayer should resemble, "Thy Will Be Done". If you have lost a loved one, it doesn't mean your prayers were unanswered. This is because we cannot fully understand God's Will or what lies beyond death in this life. The spirit of your loved one lives on.

So what is this "Spirit" that lives on? I believe spirits are born when we are born as a living human being, though already with "prior lives". The Spirit's prior lives are carried through genetic codes and, after birth, by the stories told, and the care given, to the growing child. Our Spirit grows as we grow but has an existence of its own, closely related to our learning and actions. It seems that my Spirit is connected to all other Spirits to one degree or another. There is a "Holy Spirit" which connects us all. When my body was near death my Spirit was full of life. My Spirit received the Love and Prayers for me and passed on energy and a will-to-live. That, along with excellent care, led to my survival and healing from ARDS.

We all have the inborn ability to Love and are Loved, to Pray for others and to be Prayed for by others. These are "Elements of Healing" available for free for all of us! Prayers of any type have power. We may have different religions and talk in different languages but prayer is part of every chosen belief system. And, however we visualize what happens after death, the soul of the departed person lives on in those who knew him or her. At this moment the souls of my parents live on. So do the souls of Carrie Bookless, Sheridan Alonzo, Tom Wales, Eric Gebelein and many others.

DIFFERENT VIEWS ON PRAYER

Eileen Rubin Zacharias (ERZ) is a Jewish attorney and ARDS survivor. Eileen's own encounter with ARDS and her subsequent dedication and accomplishment in establishing the ARDS Foundation USA (1), amaze me! What follows is a letter that gives a personal approach to prayer to which many people would subscribe. My views, in fact, are very close to Eileen's as we struggle with the meaning of the word "prayer" and what do we mean when we almost casually say, "I am praying for you?" Thanks to ERZ's comments on my early draft of the chapter on Prayer, I have considered her questions more carefully. Her comments and questions are so well presented in her own words -rather than mine - I am pleased to have her message printed for your interest and use. (By the way, I learned that Jewish theology teaches Jews to write"G-d" for what I would write "God".)

(1) The ARDS Foundation USA is a not for profit organization composed of a group of individuals who have been personally affected by ARDS. We are dedicated to increasing public awareness, education, and financial assistance to those engaged in medical research.
www.ardsfoundationUSAI.com

Eileen's message:

I am Jewish and believe in G-d, was bat mitzvah, raised kosher, conservative, but ended up marrying a Catholic gentleman. Even though I believe in G-d, I don't know if I believe in prayer, understand prayer, understand what its power is, feel its power... In fact, when I write to all of these people whose loved ones are in crisis, I feel sometimes that I am ill-equipped...I hate saying anything like "my prayers are with you..." even though my thoughts are and even though I would be saddened if something bad happened or happy if something positive occurred. But I usually do use those terms because I do know that for the majority of the population, those words are a great comfort to them, even when they come from a stranger and it takes nothing from me. And when these people I have corresponded with for weeks, sometimes months, have a loved one die, I find now, that the words of condolence are coming easier and I am not sure what that is saying about me either. (I hope it is not making me colder.) But, personally I have never overtly asked G-d for anything. So, when I was so very ill, just out of my coma and struggling to get off the vent but unable, it never occurred to me to ask for G-d's help. And I think somehow, when I decided to get off the vent, He must have been there with me. I was at a point where I did not care, was content not to get off, to just lay there in a bed on a vent...I tell people that getting off the vent was the hardest thing that I have ever done...harder than doing a murder jury. But I remember the day (it was a Sunday) that I made up my mind, that if I wanted to have a family, if I wanted to have children, I would have to get off this machine and out this bed and, as the doctors and therapists and my family had been telling me, walk out of this hospital. So, on Monday, when my occupational therapist, who was my own personal angel, arrived to PUSH me for the day's regime, I worked harder than I had ever and I reduced my vent settings that day and every day after that.

And when I was in my four-week coma, I was told (later) about a man who knew me from my synagogue. He used to sit near our family during the high holidays, and he learned how ill I was. He went to synagogue each morning to say the prayer for the dead for his mother who had died recently and so he told my father that he would include me in his daily prayer for the sick. After I got out of the hospital, I was told that he still included me in his prayers.

But I have to tell you that I am one of those people who have always had my doubts about prayer...

Thanks to Eileen for sharing her views on prayer. Next we have the views of my oldest son Thomas. Tom responds to an early draft of my Prayer Chapter with some very thought-provoking comments (in italics). My responses are in this font.

It is very profound to hear of your waking up and reading these 500+ cards and so forth. It is the personal aspect of this story, your story, which is the most meaningful. It is very interesting to read your account of how you changed your views on prayer, although it raises even more questions. WHY did you change your views? Why did you decide that 500+ cards stating that people were praying for you actually revealed a truth about why you recovered?

I know it's not "scientific" but I experienced the feeling that prayer was a force in my recovery when the "expert consultants" were pessimistic. Of course, this was after the fact of my recovery. So many people attest to the power of prayer, in so many religions, over so many years—who am I to deny prayer just because I can't fully explain it.

I happen to believe that the prayers did work, that they were a crucial element. I also happen to believe that perhaps a subtle aspect of your "being" or "spirit" or (sub)consciousness perhaps WAS aware of all the prayers (no physical proximity being needed - something more "psychic" for lack of a better word), and that this gave you the strength or encouragement or motivation to build upon the necessary medical assistance to pull out and recover. But why did YOU change your views? I'm very happy and moved that you did (I find "scientific materialism" in its starkest form to be philosophically very naive and ethically and emotionally somewhat bankrupt) - but WHY did you? Then again, perhaps you don't know why – you just did. No intellectual gymnastics, you just had a profound life-and-death experience and you changed. That's pretty neat too!

Regarding "God" - I'm often a bit uncomfortable hearing you talk abut "God" as it seems a bit disingenuous, in the sense that I do not think that you "believe in God" in the ways that most people do (based on years of conversations with you). It seems as if you are appropriating this word (for acceptance? for persuasion?), redefining it and then using it in your own way. You are of course entitled to do this - but I hope you clarify this up front, at the beginning of the book. Then it's FINE. But the majority of Christians, Jews, Muslims, (Hindus? New Agers?) shouldn't be led to believe that you are "speaking their language" when in fact I think that you are rather BORROWING their language. Isn't this true?

Wow! I KNOW I do not believe in God the way that most people do but I am finally able to speak about God using Christian language since this still is consistent with my beliefs and doesn't cause conflict on matters that I translate into my model. For example, I believe God is a force, not a "Him" personified, if one chooses, as a "Father." I take the Quaker view that "There is that of God in every person." I believe that "Heaven" is not a PLACE we go after death but, rather, a state of our being while alive on Earth. As to beliefs about "life after death", I'm happy to wait to find out later! (Sorry if this is irreverent or a poor joke!) We will carry on this dialogue - and "Yes," I'll "borrow" other languages to communicate. There are many ways to speak of God, Love and Peace—and Humor!

Having presented ERZ's skeptical views about prayer and TY's skepticism about my views, let's look at several interviews of others evaluation of effectiveness of prayer.

EFFECTIVENESS OF PRAYER

"Where there is no effective prayer,
life – the heart of religion –
has ceased to beat…"
Dale Turner, Seattle Times, July 28, 2001

A strong testimony on the effectiveness of prayer was sent to me by Ryan Gardner from Utah.

On April 15, 2001 Ryan was thrown out of the sunroof of a vehicle traveling over 80 mph. He had extensive injuries and after helicopter transport to the University of Utah Hospital in Salt Lake City he received emergency surgeries to pack his bleeding liver and fix his broken arm. He developed ARDS and was placed in a rotating bed. While in a coma, he recalls, "I remember feeling the presence of God and I had visions of angels. I was given the choice whether to stay alive or not … I chose to fight for life."

When the pastor of his sister's church came to the hospital for a bedside prayer, Ryan couldn't speak or open his eyes, but he remembers the overwhelming sense of power he received. Since the time of his accident he prays every day, thanking God for sparing his life. He has found a home church which he attends every Sunday. He states, "prayer saved my life".

****

With my interest in other cases showing the effectiveness of prayer, I asked Eileen Zacharias to send out a questionnaire through her network of ARDS survivors (ARDS USA). The questionnaire:

> *"To what extent do you believe that PRAYER played a role in your recovery? Please give a number from 1 to 10 where 1 equals not at all, 5 equals moderate effect, and 10 equals major effect. Please include any examples which might help others."*

Here are four responses to this questionnaire:

Dee Storey (See Dee's story in section, "Inspiring Stories")

> *I would have to say a 10. I know I was on several prayer chains - prayer chains conducted by people I'd never met and I've still to meet. I was in a drug induced coma and people who heard about my condition called others who were members of prayer chains and those prayers started for me.*
>
> *I was in a Catholic hospital when in ARDS crisis. Although I'm Jewish, a Catholic priest came to visit me every day. He was a highlight of many of my days. He would enter my room and greet me "Shalom." He would ask me if I was having a glad day, sad day, or mad day. He would select his readings from the Old Testament based on my response. He was gentle and thought provoking.*
>
> *I don't remember when I was able to think clearly enough to pray for myself. The medications at first made me really bleary in my mind. I don't remember when I began to pray for others in the ARDS community...but in praying for them, I learned a lot about myself and how much I appreciated others praying for me. I don't know to what degree prayers are efficacious in terms of physical health and recovery specifically*

68

from ARDS, but I do know that I feel a greater sense of calm when I'm praying and after I've prayed.

Dee's story indicates that worship of God need not be denominational.

****

Krissi

Krissi is an ARDS survivor living in Illinois.

I was diagnosed with ARDS when I broke out with chicken pox. I had Varicella Pneumonia, which developed quickly into ARDS. I was on the vent for 2 weeks. During that time, my fiancé and mom were by my side day and night. A priest came and prayed over me and talked to me, as well as prayed with my family. Of course, I didn't hear him and couldn't respond. He also said a prayer at Sunday mass. My fiancé's grandfather held prayer chains and said the rosary outside my ICU room. The prayers were tremendous and all over the world.

Do I think that prayer played a role in my recovery? On the scale of 1 to 10, I would say 15. If it were not for God Himself, I would not have survived and I completely believe in the power of prayer more so now than ever. My family and I thank God every day that He spared my life.

Krissi's testimony bears witness to her belief, which is similar to many other "believers".

****

Scott Bristol

Scott and I were each at Harborview Hospital in Seattle. He notes the "laying on of hands" (which is "healing touch" combined with prayer) helped him recover from ARDS.

In regards to what I think about the power of prayer I give it a 10. It was very important in my opinion. I talked to my wife and she figured about 500 to 800 people were praying for me in several different churches. A Mormon friend of mine in Richland, Washington called the church in Seattle, Washington and he came up and got together with a few other local Mormons and they performed the laying of the hands on me.

I was at Harborview, but most of the people praying for me were from the local churches in the tri-cities area of eastern Washington. I was at Harborview in January of 2000 for 7 weeks. I was on the vent for 6 weeks and coded 3 times. I also had an out-of-body experience. I am much closer to God these days than I was before this and I am still trying to figure out what He wants me to do, I figure if He saved me 3 times He's got to have plans for me. I just don't know what His plans are yet. But I guess I am one of the lucky ones. Most people were on the vent a lot less then I was and have a lot of after effects. I have hardly any. I just use an inhaler every great once in a while.

I don't understand "out of body experience", but others have referred to it, so I guess I still have more to learn.

****

Dan Bennett

Dan is another ARDS survivor deemed to be a "miracle man"

I was on the vent for about a week or so. I was supposed to be in the hospital for 3 to 4 months; then I was supposed to be at home for another 2 to 3 months recovering. I was out of the hospital in two weeks. Loyola called me the "Miracle" patient and actually had a symposium on my rapid recovery. The official hospital reason for my rapid recovery was "Divine

Intervention".

 While in my coma, my father would lead the family (circled around my bed) in prayer. Sometimes a priest would come in as well. We are Roman Catholic.

 I would not be here if it were not for the power of prayer. I am 40 years old, the father of five, and a full time police officer (and part time stand up comedian / singer).

Dan and I met on the internet. I look forward to meeting with him for a few jokes and songs – hopefully with no police action!

Although some may be skeptical of prayer chains, I am impressed with the number of people – some not even knowing me – who prayed for me as part of a "Prayer Chain". Obviously, any number of people telling their story about the power of prayer does not "prove" that prayer works via God – or any other system. Stories do, however, capture our attention and beg for explanation. For whatever prayer is worth, I'm alive today to read articles such as the following, which I will share with you.

SELECTED ARTICLES ON PRAYER & SPIRITUALITY IN MEDICINE

 Simply by "random reading" I have run across a number of articles related to prayer and spirituality in medicine. I will share some of the points in these articles, which may be of interest to you.

 In an article, *"Can Prayer Heal?"* in The Saturday Evening Post – December 2001, Jeanie Davis describes a pilot study on the effects of "distant care and the outcome of patients undergoing high risk procedures". Dr. Mitchell Krucoff, a cardiologist at Duke University School of Medicine is reported as studying prayer at a distance in a study which will enroll 1500 patients undergoing coronary angioplasty at nine centers around the country. Patients are being randomly assigned to four study groups. In addition to standard medical care, Group 1 will be prayed for; Group 2 will receive bedside spiritual therapy and relaxation; Group 3 will receive both of these;

Group 4 will receive none of the extra spiritual therapies. As witnessed by The Saturday Evening Post article, there is a public interest in spiritual therapy and prayer in Medicine.

Even getting away in an airplane does not free you from articles about *"Spiritual Healing"* as in the November 15, 2000 issue of American Way. The article discusses a study by the American Psychological Association which studied the degree of religious involvement. Those who scored higher in religious interests had a 29% higher chance of survival than those with a less active spiritual life. It was speculated that those who pray or attend church may be less likely to be obese, to smoke cigarettes, to use drugs or alcohol. The article goes on to discuss approaches to prayer, meditation, yoga, and community worship.

The Reader's Digest, October, 1999 (which frequently publishes articles on religious topics) published an article, *"Faith Is Powerful Medicine"* by Phyllis McIntosh abstracted from *"Remedy"*. She notes that,

> *"Most of us have heard of cases in which someone, seemingly by sheer faith and will, has miraculously recovered from a terminal illness or survived far longer than doctors thought possible."*

The article sites several of more than 30 studies that have found a connection between spiritual or religious commitment and longer life. It also mentions controversial studies suggesting that prayer can influence everything, from the growth of bacteria in a lab to healing wounds in mice.

The article continues by reporting that at a national medical meeting in 1996 a survey of 269 family physicians showed that 99% believe that religious beliefs contribute to healing and 63% indicated that God had intervened in their own medical conditions.

The Reader's Digest is one of my favorite publications, combining humor with spiritual and other relevant articles.

In the medical arena, The New England Journal of Medicine, June 22, 2000, has an article by Richard Sloan, *"Should Physicians Prescribe Religious Activities?"* He quips that "medicine of the future may be prayer and Prozac". He indicates that more than 30 U. S.

medical schools offer courses in religious spirituality and health. Ph.D. Doctors Sloan and Bagiella, with seven associates, provide an interesting discussion and 29 references, but don't come to any strikingly clear answers to their question. In their conclusions they say, "Because the question of a link between religion and health care is so controversial, we must continue to address it with discussions that cross disciplinary and specialty lines."

Continuing on in the medical arena, Dr. Larry Dossey has a "commentary" in the June 26, 2000 issue of Arch Intern Med, titled *"Prayer and Medical Science – a Commentary on the Prayer Study by Harris et al and a Response to Critics"*. Dossey compares disbelief in the power of prayer to disbelief in gravity before Newton in the 17th century.

> *"Today we are as baffled by the remote effects of prayer as Newton's critics were by the distant effects of gravity."*

Dossey defends skepticism as "an invaluable component of scientific progress" but warns that it can "shade into a type of dogmatic materialism" that excludes intercessory prayer in principle. Forty-six references are included with this excellent commentary.

Dossey's address and email are published as 878 Paseo del Sur, Santa Fe, NM 87501, (email: ldossey@ix.netcom.com)

The opinions of all the persons above don't matter at all. What matters is YOUR opinion! Nevertheless, there is a certain enchantment in hearing what celebrities think about any subject, including prayer. Just remember Fred Allen's quip:

> *"A celebrity is a person who works hard all his life to become known, then wears dark glasses to avoid being recognized."*

So, take off your dark glasses and read "Powerful Prayers" by Larry King.

"POWERFUL PRAYERS"

*"Pray to God
but continue to row to shore"*
Russian Proverb

The book, "Powerful Prayers", written by **Larry King** with **Rabbi Irwin Katsof**, published in 1998, (by Renaissance Books) is a remarkable series of interviews with some of today's well-known personalities who reveal their views on prayer and religion.

Over 85% of all Americans claim that they pray, yet prayer is unique for each individual, even when part of a group. Rabbi Katsof notes that prayer is easy and prayer is difficult ... easy because it is a conversation, and difficult because you must pay close attention to your words and thoughts. "Prayer connects you to your true self."

Country music legend Willie Nelson believes songs can be prayers and is quoted, "prayer has kept me from killing myself". Folk singer Pete Seeger told Larry that songs were prayers, and Larry indicates that he started to understand that "a song is a pretty good foundation upon which to build a prayer". Some songs are more obvious than others such as "You'll Never Walk Alone" and "I Say a Little Prayer For You", and "What a Wonderful World", and "I Believe". I've already indicated that music is one of the six "elements of healing" that aided my recovery from ARDS.

King relates his interview of Anthony Robbins who tells the story of Howard, who had a heart attack during one of Robbins' classes. When the EMTs arrived, and used the defibrillator, they declared after 10 minutes, "He's gone". Robbins asserted, "You are not giving up on this man". A physician attending the seminar said, "You're wasting your time – there's nothing that can be done. The man has been dead for 45 minutes." CPR was continued en route to the hospital and until the doctor was seen. Howard had a pulse and soon thereafter the doctor said, "He's alive". The physician in the seminar, who had declared Howard dead, wept when he was told of Howard's survival, as he thought about all the people he might have saved after having declared them dead.

I can identify with being written off as "hopeless" by some physicians, while other physicians and my family did not give up hope.

Who can tell the power of thousands of prayers for my recovery? My recovery is considered a miracle … outside the bounds of medical probability. The lesson is, "don't give up hope prematurely. Where there is life there is hope!"

"There are no hopeless situations …
only people who give up hope!"

In his book, King tells his own story noting his father died of a heart attack at age 44. King, himself, had experienced some of the "miracles of modern medicine", including an angioplasty and quintuple coronary bypass surgery. Subsequently, in June of 1997, he was told he would need to have a repeat angioplasty. The night before this procedure, his fiancé, Shawn Southwick, "a devout Mormon", led a group in prayer for Larry. Larry joined the prayer circle and bowed his head "out of respect". Larry notes "I'm still in neutral, but I hope to hell Shawn is in drive". He goes on to say that he did feel a peace after that prayer, and that the angioplasty went fine. On September 4th 1997, two days before the wedding, another artery was clogged and he was told he had to return to New York for more surgery. On September 5th, at 6 a.m. he and Shawn were married in his hospital room, just an hour before he was flown back to New York for his angioplasty.

King has started a Cardiac Foundation with an annual fund raiser to help those who can't afford heart surgery. King's foundation is non-denominational and he quotes Bob Hope as saying:

"I do benefits for all religions.
I'd hate to blow the hereafter
on a technicality."

Larry King quotes Howard Schultz, founder of Starbucks as saying "I prayed to God on an ongoing basis about the opportunity to build a company that valued the human spirit … not only about building profit but about being the kind of person who does the right thing."

J. W. Marriott, Chairman and CEO of Marriott International, believes in praying for assistance, not necessarily for end results. King observes that Marriott, like his wife Shawn, is Mormon and notes that, "Jews and Mormons have a lot in common. Both were wandering tribes in search of a permanent home. The Jews went east; the Mormons went west. We got the desert and they got Utah!"

The role of prayer in medical care is largely anecdotal, but King interviewed one doctor, Larry Dossey, who has written on scientific studies of prayer. King asks Dossey, "How do you think prayer works in healing?" Dossey's answer indicates, "we are going to have to rethink the nature of consciousness", making consciousness a property of more than the brain. Dossey sees consciousness as a property of the universe akin to matter and energy, and able to have affects at a distance such as we see in prayer. Prayer is universal and there never has been a culture without some form of prayer. "The idea that we have to keep science and spirituality apart is an idea whose time has come and gone."

King asks Dossey if there is a particular kind of prayer that works best. Dossey replies that he doesn't think it makes a bit of difference how people pray, as long as they pray with a sense of love, compassion and empathy coming from the heart.

Prayer is a choice and without choice we can go nowhere. To paraphrase, a story that Irwin Katsof tells:

> *A man on a desert half way between two water sources dies of thirst because he is unable to choose which way to go!*

King's book ends with an epilogue by Katsof, closing with a beautiful prayer:

> *May the Almighty grant us and our children the wisdom to live our lives to the utmost and may he bless us with good health, wisdom, and happiness."*

LARRY DOSSEY'S STUDIES ON PRAYER

The question is, "Do prayers like this really work?" Dr. Larry Dossey reports studies of prayer in his books *"Healing Words"* (1993) and

"Reinventing Medicine" (1999), but as Dossey quotes C.S. Lewis as saying:

> *"...however badly needed a good book on prayer is, I shall never try to write it ... For me to offer the world instruction about prayer would be impudence."*

In spite of Lewis' warning, Dossey's books present evidence that prayer is a force as real as gravity and as visible as light. Dossey's concept of the *"nonlocal mind"* relates to interaction of minds at a distance similar to distant interactions of electrons. Dossey states:

> *"Many studies reveal that healing can be achieved at a distance by directing loving and compassionate thoughts, intentions, and prayers to others who may even be unaware of these efforts..."*

Dossey discusses the evolution of medical thinking to the current era, conceptualizing both individual and collective consciousness – i.e. both local and nonlocal being. A simple example of nonlocality is where the nurses or doctors' mood or mental state has a direct effect on the patient's clinical course. I believe that positive moods of anyone around comatose patients have a beneficial effect. In addition to the stories in this book, there are numerous other cases where prayer and positive attitudes have seemed to lead to good outcomes in critically ill patients.

Readers interested in prayer as an element of healing are well-advised to read Larry Dossey's books *"Healing Words"* and *"Reinventing Medicine"*.

HOW PRAYER HEALS

Readers who are interested in a practical guide to prayer and healing may be interested in the book by Walter Weston, "How Prayer Heals". Weston notes,

"Prayers for the sick – any place on earth – take on universal characteristics that transcend religious beliefs"

This is a book that gives eighteen reasons for using spoken prayer, asserting silent prayer for the sick is not as effective as praying out loud. Weston says that the person being healed does not need to believe in God, but must have two characteristics: 1) a desire to become well; and 2) trust in healing prayer. The person offering healing prayer need have no qualifications other than a loving concern.

Weston reviews the work of Doctors Herbert Benson and Bernie Siegel. Faith in prayer, as well as faith in physicians, medications, and procedures opens the possibility of healing. Siegel's "exceptional cancer patients" recover from terminal cancer associated with faith that a change in lifestyle will make them well. There appears to be agreement that negative, cynical beliefs in an ill person reduce the chance of healing and may negate any effects of prayer.

Weston assures us:
"A pleasant surprise awaits you.
As you journey on your path of prayer for wholeness,
you will be blessed far beyond what you had ever hoped."

A PERSONAL HISTORY OF PRAYER

"Now I lay me down to sleep,
I pray the Lord my soul to keep.
If I should die before I wake,
I pray the Lord my soul to take."

This prayer recited with my parents when I was about 2 years old is still fixed in my memory 66 years later. I now have some reservations about focusing a child on dying before waking, but I've never had any sleep problems.

Our Father, which art in heaven ...
... thy will be done

The "Lord's Prayer" was the second prayer I learned to recite, sometimes with "forgive us our debts" and sometimes with "forgive us our trespasses". Although all of this prayer has meaning, I believe the most important request is *"thy will be done"*. I still love this prayer and particularly like it in its musical rendition, combining the elements of prayer and music.

My next paradigm shift in prayer came in medical school when I joined the Religious Society of Friends (Quakers), practicing meditation and silent prayer. This is still my primary practice today. Although I am comfortable with spoken "grace" at festivities, I am most comfortable with "a moment of silence".

In terms of prayer as "an element of healing", I am convinced that the strength and number of prayers were fundamental in my recovery and return to medical practice. I also pray silently for my patients who are in difficult circumstances.

SUMMARY

*"Prayer ... properly understood and applied
is the most potent instrument of action."*
Gandhi (1948)

Related to "Love", "Prayer" is one of the most important elements of healing "Beyond Medicine". I believe my own survival was related not only to the excellent medical care, but also to the extent of love and prayer for me.

There are differing views on prayers as an element of healing "Beyond Medicine", as told in the stories of individuals in this chapter. My own belief is that no one model is "right".

Everyone has his own experience with prayer.

The writings of two "Larrys" – King and Dossey – provide intellectual stimulation on the topic of prayer. King's interviews of celebrities, and Rabbi Irwin Katsof's insights, provide provocative thoughts on "the power of prayer". Dossey's discussion of the "nonlocal mind" gives a model for how prayer works.

REFERENCES

The ARDS Foundation, www.ardsfoundationusa.com

Holden Village www.holdenvillage.org (See footnote for address)

Dossey, Larry, "Healing Words", 1993, HarperSanFrancisco

Dossey, Larry, "Prayer Is Good Medicine", 1996, HarperSanFrancisco

Dossey, Larry, "Reinventing Medicine", 1999, HarperSanFrancisco

Frankl, Victor E. "Man's Search for Meaning", 1959, Simon & Schuster

King, Larry, "Powerful Prayers", 1998, Renaissance Books

Weston, Walter "How Prayer Heals, 1998, Hampton Roads"

APPENDIX

Sometimes we can be overwhelmed by the chain letters that assault us by email. Every once in awhile one of these is worth noting and passing on. Here are highlights from one, the author which is unknown to me, which speaks of an attitude towards God and our prayers to God:

> *I asked God to take away my pain. God said, "No.*
> *It is not for me to take away, But for you to give it up."*

> *I asked God to give me happiness. God said, "No.*
> *I give you blessings, Happiness is up to you."*

> *I asked God for everything that I might enjoy life. God said,*
> *"No. I will give you life, It's up to you to enjoy."*

This prayer reminds us not to ask God for things that are our responsibility.

The next email wonder is attributed to The Dalai Lama message on the millennium, entitled "Instructions for Life". The message reads:

Take into account that great love and great achievements involve great risk.

When you lose, don't lose the lesson

Follow the three R's: Respect for self ... Respect for others ...Responsibility for all your actions.

Remember that not getting what you want is sometimes a wonderful stroke of luck.

Learn the rules so you know how to break them properly.

Don't let a little dispute injure great friendship.

When you realize you've made a mistake, take immediate steps to correct it.

Spend some time alone every day.

Open your arms to change, but don't let go of your values.

Remember that silence is sometimes the best answer.

Live a good honorable life. Then when you get older and think back, you'll be able to enjoy it a second time.

A loving atmosphere in your home is the foundation for your life.

In disagreements with loved ones, deal only with the current situation. Don't bring up the past.

Share your knowledge. It's a way to achieve immortality.

Be gentle with the earth.

Once a year, go some place you've never been before.

Remember that the best relationship is one in which your love for each other exceeds your need for each other.

Judge your success by what you had to give up in order to get it.

Approach love and cooking with reckless abandon.

[i] *Holden Village was built at the site of an abandoned copper mine at the northwest end of Lake Chelan in central Washington. Summer programs feature a wide range of discussions led by faculty from many places. For more information see the offline website www.holdenvillage.org or write to Holden Village, HC00 Stop 2, Chelan, Washington, 98816-9769. They have no e-mail or telephone - a delightful freedom! This magical place is full of "Holy Hilarity" and freedom from stress that comes from Wilderness Mountain living with a basic, natural diet.*

TOUCH - WITHOUT WHICH LIFE CEASES

Whereas love and prayer touched me at a spiritual and psychological level, plain old ordinary touch was an essential element of healing for me. I needed touch as much as a baby needs touch. In fact, I learned in medical school that many babies died from being raised in sterile bassinettes so that their mothers could work in wartime factories. The babies were barely touched and many died of a condition termed "anaclitic depression".

Good parenting involves a lot of touch of the growing child, and the untouched child cries loudly to express his/her need. Babies cry out for touch and are soothed when held and rocked. Breastfeeding or closely holding a baby being fed by a bottle is one of the early examples of touch as a love and healing force.

The growing child is taught that "a kiss will make it better", and being held is the remedy for minor falls, bumps and bangs.

The teenager or adult suffering emotional trauma is comforted by being held. One of the things that we say to people who have suffered a loss is, "stay in touch". Here "touch" is a metaphor for keeping communication intact, but how appropriate.

Touch as an element in healing is also extremely important for persons with medical problems. Unfortunately, doctors and nurses touch patients much less than in the past. The increased use of technology including Xrays, ECG's, blood tests, CT scans, ultrasound studies, etc. has decreased the significance of the "physical examination" which requires the use of touch.

Possibly the increased popularity of chiropractors and massage therapists is a result of decreased touch in traditional care. The touch of chiropractors and massage therapists is, in itself, therapeutic. Physicians and nurses could choose to use more simple touch as a therapeutic tool. Touch is a communication of caring and expresses a connection between the caregiver and the patient. Family and friends also communicate by touch, particularly if the patient is in a coma or heavily sedated.

Touch for reassurance may be one of the most overlooked elements of healing. From a handshake to a friendly pat on the back or touch to the forearm, there can be a lot of positive, healing messages transmitted to the patient from family, friends, or professionals.

In my own experience as a patient of ARDS, I found that touch by my family and caregivers became something that I craved. I'm particularly grateful to Sandy Sallee, LMT, for providing massage therapy in our home during my recovery. Massage of painful and stiff areas helped relieve symptoms. However, I recall one occasion when I asked a nurse to massage the palm of my hand to relieve a painful spasm in that area. She informed me, "Sorry, that's not in my job description. Would you like a pain pill?" As a physician for over 40 years, I have seen the role of massage by nurses become less and less part of their "job description." I suggest it's time to reverse history and restore massage as a more central part of nursing care. Wouldn't it be nice to have less paperwork and more "touchwork"?

Massage of the lower legs is useful in promoting circulation and reducing the risk of blood clots. I believe there is far too much concern about releasing clots by massage. Pulmonary emboli (blood clots to the lungs) are more likely to be prevented than caused by massage.

Passive range of motion and massage are very important to prevent stiffness and contractures (fixed bending) in bedridden patients. This includes shoulders, elbows, wrists, fingers, hips, knees, toes and ankles. In my case, I developed contractures of my fingers in spite of regular therapy by my family while I was comatose. Now that I am out of a coma, I can work on my own physical therapy and my fingers are straightening out. One of the consequences of my stiff fingers is difficulty using the computer mouse. I have adapted by reversing the left and right click buttons on the mouse. Also, typing and writing are very difficult for me, but are gradually improving.

Some forms of touch among males appear humorous to an outside observer. "High-fives" along with other hand slapping rituals, shoulder punching, fist bonking, back patting, fanny slapping, chest bucking, and head butting are all symbolic forms of touch communication. Even hugging is often seen in athletic events!

Hugging is a form of therapy that family and friends can give to their loved ones. Hugging is another area of healing touch beyond medicine. Hugging, like massage, has decreased in medicine due in part to time constraints and also to fear of inappropriate contact and sexual harassment liability. I still hug my patients when it is clear that a hug will be appropriately received. In the same sense, I appreciated hugs when I was recovering from ARDS – and still find hugs a healing force.

In an era of high-tech medicine it is important not to lose touch with "hands on" traditions. Massage is one tradition which utilizes a variety of techniques. Some of these techniques are:

Acupressure	*Polarity*
Stress Reduction	*Chair massage*
Reflexology	*Swedish*
Cranial Sacral	*Rolfing*
Therapeutic Touch	*Deep tissue*
Shiatsu	*Thai Massage*
Facial massage	*Lomilomi*
Myofascial	*Hellerwork*

A search on the web for "Therapeutic Massage" brought up over 201,000 hits. Interestingly, the first listing was Charles Stanley's "In Touch Ministries".

As another outcome of our internet research, we learned of "Touch Research Institutes". We are told that the first TRI was established in 1992 by Tiffany Field, Ph.D. at the University of Miami School of Medicine[i]. This TRI is claimed to be the first center in the world devoted solely to touch in the field of medicine.

There are training programs in massage offered at many sites around the country. There are also varying certifying programs to become an "LMT" (Licensed Massage Therapist). A registry of massage sites and therapists is provided on the internet[ii].

There are various certifying boards for massage therapists (and many techniques as listed above). There is a National Certification Board for Therapeutic Massage and Bodywork, headquartered in McLean, VA[iii].

One of the items on the massage smorgasbord is "Healing Touch", which is a technique difficult to visualize by those of us who are conventionally trained professionals. "Healing Touch" is an energy (biofield) therapy that encompasses a group of non-invasive techniques that utilize the hands to clear, energize, and balance the human and environmental energy fields. More information can be obtained from their website[iv]. It's claimed that "hands-on touch modalities are used by more than 30,000 nurses in hospitals each year, and that the procedures are documented as legitimate medical techniques".

Another technique is the "laying on of hands" with spiritual communication for physical healing, which is practiced by many believers.

For all I know, some of these therapies may have been used on me while I was in a coma, but I must admit that I lack full awareness and information on these alternative health care methods. There is a great need for more research and teaching related to these methods. I do know that the touch and muscle massage I received while I was in the hospital, and during my rehabilitation phase were important elements of healing beyond the medical care I received.

Beyond high-tech medicine there are basic "hands on" elements of healing. Hands may still help healing. We should touch each patient at every level - mental, physical and spiritual.

SUMMARY

Let's keep in touch with touch.

Appendix: Multiple Meanings of Touch

Keep in touch (communicate)
His words touch you (create emotion)
He touched on the issue (hit lightly)
Put the touch on someone (ask for a donation)
Washington touches Canada (borders)
No one was touched by the explosion (wounded)
A little touched (crazy)
Touch down (airplane) *vs. Touchdown* (football)
A good touch (physician, chef, musician)
A touch of pepper (a little bit)
Touch and go (uncertain)
Therapeutic touch (massage)
Healing touch (hand contact for healing)
Etc.

[i] Touch Research Institutes
University of Miami School of Medicine
P O Box 016820
Miami FL 33101
305-243-6781
www.miami.edu/touch-research/history.html

[ii] www.massageregister.com

[iii] National Certification Board for Therapeutic Massage and Bodywork
8201 Greensboro Drive, Suite 300
McLean, VA 22102
1-800-296-0664
www.ncbtmb.com/

[iv] www.healingtouch.net/

HUMOR – HOW HUMOR HEALS

"I don't mind dying - I just don't want to be there when it happens"
Woody Allen

"The first thing I do in the morning is read the Obituary Column. If I'm not in it I fix a cup of coffee and get ready for the day."
George Burns

The search on the Internet on Google indicated 9,320,000 references were available on Humor and 479,000 on "Humor and Medicine"

I see no sense in losing one's sense of humor just because the situation is serious. Humor is an element of healing that was very important in my recovery from my ARDS. Of course I was in a coma for the first 32 days or so of my hospital adventure, so I wasn't exactly what you would call a stand up comic! Never the less, my family realized the value I placed on humor and were able to laugh and play games to ease their tension in the waiting room. I am told that the game of "Celebrities" was a big laugh getter, but I wasn't there to play with them.

After my transfer to Harborview, when I was awake but still bed-bound, I do remember the reawakening of my sense of humor coincident with my sense of bladder fullness after my urinary catheter was removed. I played games with the nurses who had to measure my vital signs (temperature, heart rate, respiratory rate, blood pressure), blood oxygen saturation and urine volume. I pretended to know the numbers before they took the measurements and we were all amazed and amused at the accuracy of my guesses. For example, I was surprised at how close I came on urine volumes.

One event where humor prevailed over modesty happened when I was awake but too weak to feed myself or move in bed. The nurse caring for me seemed younger than my daughter yet aware I was in pain after she rolled me over in bed. Struggling with how to say the source of my pain, I finally said, "Would you please untuck me?" She gave me a bewildered look until obliging my request with a smile when I explained, "I'm lying on my private parts - would you please untuck my scrotum?"

Another example of "urinary humor" came at 7:05 a.m. one day when I pushed the call button to make a request. "What would you like?" the clerk inquired. "I need a urinal" I replied ... "Sorry, the nurses are in Report," I was told ... "If they don't come now they'll have something to report alright," I warned ... "Someone will be there by 7:15," I was assured ... At 7:30 I called to report that the Weather Report was for "Showers and very wet". At 7:31 the forecast came true, and when a nurse appeared 2 minutes later I reassured her of her job security for changing bed linen...and told her to record a urine output of 310 cc! (I stifled my suggestion that she see what it feels like to lie on liquid-laden linen.) ... So much for the sacred position of "Nursing Report".

Not all of my humor experiences were centered in my body. I particularly appreciated the more than 500 cards I received, many of which were humorous. My family prepared a poster collage and others enjoyed these cards as I did.

Then there was the visit of a group of Seafair Clowns who managed to find a parking place for their clown vehicle on the sidewalk and somehow or other joked their way through nurse guards to appear in full clown garb at my bedside. In addition to being great clowns, these guys were also great friends, as I myself have been a Seafair Clown for over 20 years playing the character "Dr. Quack" ... "The Quack Is Back!" they proclaimed ... "Some guys will do anything to get a little attention," I was jibed. (Parenthetically I recovered enough in the next few months to join my fellow clowns in the year 2000 Seattle Seafair celebrations – though mostly as a "fire truck clown" riding on the clown fire truck vehicle.)

Just as Norman Cousins did, I watched humorous videos, listened to comedy tapes and read funny material as a form of "Humor Therapy". The ensuing laughter was healing to my mind and body (as it had been to Cousins).

The attendees of the Year 2000 Conference on Humor and Creativity held in Saratoga Springs, New York sent me an amazing humorous greeting while I was still in the hospital. On two large sheets of butcher paper they inscribed messages of humor and good will, which brought laughter to my lungs and tears to my eyes. I sent my thanks to Joel Goodman and Margie Ingram – founders and coordinators of the Humor Project, which organizes the annual conference each spring. I had attended almost every conference up to the year of my ARDS and have attended each conference since then. In addition to annual conferences, the Humor Project has a catalog of humor resources and a speaker's bureau. The annual conferences held in April each year have included a number of "big name" humorists. Naming a few from the conferences I have attended: Steve Allen, Red Skelton, Victor Borge, the Smothers Brothers, Jay Leno and others. Write the Humor Project, Inc. at 480 Broadway, Suite 210, Saratoga Springs, NY 12866, or visit their web site: www.HumorProject.com, or phone at 518-587-8770.

"A smile is the shortest distance between two people."
Victor Borge:

"There are three things which are real:
God, human folly, and laughter.
The first two are beyond our comprehension, so
we must do what we can with the third."
John F. Kennedy:

Another valuable humor resource is the AATH – American Association for Therapeutic Humor (222 S. Meramec, Suite 303, St. Louis, MO 63105, phone 314-863-6232). Individuals active with AATH include Patty Wooten, Karyn Buxman and others. Clown Nurse Patty Wooten can be reached at: Jest For the Health Of It, P O Box 4040, Davis, CA 95617, phone 916-758-3826, email: pwooten@mother.com, and web site: www.mother.com/JestHome.

Another humorous speaker who teaches how to use humor in the workplace, is Patt Schwab, PhD., an active member in NSA – National Speakers Association. Patt's talks include "When Hell Freezes Over – Ice Skate! – Coping with Change and Adversity". She quotes Charles Darwin: "It's not the strongest of the species that survives, nor the most intelligent, but the one most responsive to change". Patt can be reached at FUNdamentally Speaking, 9401 – 45th Ave. NE, Seattle, WA 98115, phone (207-525-1031, email: pattschwab@aol.com.

Humor opens our minds to creativity and change and has a

profound influence on survival and health.

Another journal which I have enjoyed is "Humor and Health Journal" published by Joseph R. Dunn, PhD. He quotes Mark Twain:

"Humor is mankind's greatest blessing".

A friend I made at the Humor and Creativity Conference in Saratoga Springs, Al Clemens from Anchorage, Alaska, says "Your smile is said to be one of the very best of dress one can wear in society ...keep smiling." Al quotes Garrison Keillor:

"Humor is not a trick, not jokes.
Humor is a presence in the world ... like grace ...
And shines on everybody."

Al can be reached at The Kindness Industry, 2515 Ingra Street, Anchorage, AK 99508, phone 907-272-5247, email: inspirational@gci.net.

There is another valuable resource related to humor, which was introduced to me after my ARDS hospitalization. This is the "World Laughter Tour" organized by Steve Wilson and his associates. (World Laughter Tour, 1159 South Creekway Court, Columbus, OH 43230, or call 1-800-NOW-LAFF, or visit www.WorldLaughterTour.com) One of the major teachings is that laughter is not the same as humor. Babies and young children laugh out of sheer delight, whereas most adults, as they grow older, tend to laugh less and less. On the other hand, laughter can be a learned skill and be part of health and healing.

Laughter was first taken seriously in 1978 when Norman Cousins wrote his book "Anatomy of an Illness". This is a classic work describing Cousins use of comic videos to reduce pain through laughter. After a period of laughter, there was an even longer period of pain-free relaxation. He said laughter was an effective exercise for health, termed "inner jogging".

The "Laughter Clubs Movement" was started by Dr. Madan Kataria, a native of India, whose book, Laugh for No Reason", was published in 1999 by Madhuri International (email: laugh@vsnl.com). Steve Wilson visited Kataria in Mumbai, India and initiated the World

Laughter Tour starting in the U.S.A. in 1999. The major discovery, which forms the base of this movement, is that humor not only leads to laughter, but laughter also leads to developing a sense of humor and laughter can be isolated from humor. A child does not laugh because he has a sense of humor, but laughs because it is his nature to be joyful. Graduates of Wilson's Laughter Club programs are designated as CLL's – Certified Laughter Leaders, capable of leading group exercises which result in laughter. "We are paying a heavy price for taking life too seriously, and now the time has come to take laughter seriously." In the 1950s a study showed people laughed 18 minutes a day, and by 1999 they laughed less than 6 minutes a day. Children laugh more than 300 times a day and adults only 15 times in the average day.

Sometimes I surprise myself with my "Patch Adams humor-behavior!" In my early years as a physician I was called to the University Hospital's medical ward for admission of an 82-year-old woman with possible pneumonia. The nurses warned me that she was a "real witch" and as mean-tempered and nasty as they'd ever seen. As I came to her doorway, sure enough she had her head off the pillow and was glowering nastily at me as if to say, "Don't you dare come in here!" I dropped my chin and walked slowly in her room, pulled back the blanket and laid down beside her, saying, "I've had a very tiring day, Mam…do you mind if I rest a moment before I do your admission history and exam?" Her response - to the amazement of the nurses standing in the doorway -was to pat my head on her shoulder, comforting me with, "There, there, young man—you just rest awhile before you do what you need to do!" From then on her care was easy - for the nurses as well as her doctors! Humor, mixed with caring, is more effective then a powerful drug!

When I was in a coma, on a ventilator in the first month of my ARDS, I'm told my sister, Nancy, used a humor technique of "Playful kidding" which elicited a faint smile and (Who Knows?) may have motivated my recovery. By way of background, Nancy and I, as children, slept in bedrooms at opposite ends of a hall which had one hall light with a switch at each end. She wanted the light ON and I wanted if OFF. We engaged in a "battle of the switches" until a parent intervened, generally taking her side since she was four years younger. Now jump ahead about 60 years and hear her speak clearly in my ear, even with my coma, "When you recover you can have the hall light on if you want it my way - or OFF if that's what YOU choose!" I chose to have my "life-light" ON and the hall light off.

Humor helped my family to lighten the load of endless hours of bedside vigil and prayer. I'm told that they knew I wanted them to laugh - and they did, over life's daily sillinesses. And they played laughter-inducing games such as "Celebrities", introduced by my son, Bob, who is an actor in New York. Laughter emerges as teams try to guess the name of the celebrity (Sports, TV, movies, politics, etc) from clues given (with rules) by one of the game players.

Ninety-two days in the hospital doesn't seem like quite as deep a dent in the days of your life if you are in a coma for 40 and have humor, touch, music, pets to help - along with needed drugs from sensitive doctors and nurses. I admit I was a bit discouraged when my trach tube was finally taken out after over 60 days. "Why not happy?" you ask. When I asked "How long will I need to cover the hole in my neck to talk?" I was told, "Not very long." "How long is 'Not very long' ?" I inquired…"Oh, not over two weeks, probably" was the response. Then I was depressed. Seeing no immediate humor to help, I opted for a nap. When I awoke 2 hours later the hole in my neck was closed and I could talk again - without a thumb over a hole in my neck. NOW I can see the humor of it all!

Humor may be realized through seeing life from a different perspective which we may call "paradoxical". What I mean by "paradoxical perspective" is the ability to see the opposite meaning of life situations so that there is no "bad news" - just "new challenges." As Oscar Wilde said on his deathbed as he gazed up at the wallpaper, "That wallpaper is awful—one of us has got to go!"

"Jokes" are only part of what we consider humor and are seen as "funny" (or not) due to a surprising or paradoxical twist at the end. Most of Humor, however, relates to our every-day attitude to life's experiences. Someone with a "Good sense of Humor" finds laughter and a sense of play in moment-to-moment events.

During my post-coma "rehabilitation" I had a variety of "T parties"—PT, OT, RT, and ST to name them by their abbreviations for Physical Therapy, Occupational Therapy, Recreational Therapy and Social Therapy. None of them did what their name suggested.

PT worked on getting me to get in and out of bed or a chair and, later, to push a wheelchair with assistance and - in graduate training as an outpatient after the3rd month of hospital care - to walk a few steps. PT, in short, was LT - Leg Therapy. I was taught so well that I still rock forward three times, counting aloud, putting my feet back and head forward (like I should fall on my face) whenever I get out of a deep chair or off a toilet. So, thanks, PT - I have yet to be stuck on a toilet seat (or need to be untucked!).

Now "OT" has to do with your HANDS and nothing to do with your occupation, or how you occupy yourself. You'd be surprised at the humor created by weak hands! No modesty works when you can't feed yourself, shave your face, pick your nose, wipe your assorted parts, work your zipper, button or unbutton, scratch wherever, tuck and untuck, etc.. I tell you it's one thing to need help with a tuck and still another with a scratch! Oh, well, at least males have no bras or periods to contend with...

RT – Recreational Therapy – should have been called TT — Trip Therapy – in reference to the trips they took us on outside of the hospital to readapt us to places like pizza parlors, museums and parks.

ST – Social Therapy may have had to do with ST = Sexual Therapy or other such social hard issues or adjustments following discharge from the hospital. Fitting into society again following ARDS may present a number of challenges. ST could also be seen as FT = Freudian Therapy. I suppose that is what ST is supposed to help with.

Another T should be MT = Massage Therapy, one of the most important elements of healing. From the laying on of hands to deep tissue massage, there are numerous variations of MT which are valuable tools for healing. Since the mind and body are connected, MT is also Mind Therapy.

Let's not forget AT = Animal Therapy, which is fully discussed in the chapter on PT = Pet Therapy!

And MT = Music Therapy also has its own chapter, not to be confused with MT discussed above.

Finally, last but not least, is HT = Humor Therapy, which also has its own chapter (this one!).

A physician can choose to present the same "facts" as. *"Too bad...you are going to need coronary bypass surgery..."* or as *"The good news is that you have a problem which can be fixed by surgery..."* The patient can see the paradox in "good news" in the second message but is left with a positive outlook in contrast to the first message.

Humor leads to a positive outlook which leads to a positive outcome. Death itself is not a defeat but can be seen as a rescue from suffering or as a "moving on" to another world.

Along with tears there can be laughter at a funeral which celebrates the life (while mourning the death) of a loved one. Carrie Bookless, whose story is told in Section III of this book, anticipating her possible demise, specified that there be no funeral but instead that there be a Celebration Party. After her tragic death her wish was met and we all recalled Carrie and her sense of humor. Her happy spirit lives on.

If there is already an alphabet soup of "T's" why not HT = Humor Therapy? I place such a high value on humor that I make it one of the primary prerequisites for people that I hire or surround myself with. Moreover, I make it a goal to have some humor and laughter as part of each patient encounter. In my clinic, for example, I often open the closed door to an exam room and enter singing a song. I try to make my first comment or question something totally irrelevant to medical problems. I like to use humorous nicknames to break down barriers and "white coat hypertension" and – as a patient myself – I appreciate doctors, nurses, and staff members who relate to me with a sense of humor. Humor is therapy and Humor Therapy is an important adjunct to traditional medical, surgical, psychological, etc. invasions.

A "sense of humor" may be partly inborn, but is largely learned, practiced, and developed by choice. "If the world gives you a lemon – make lemonade."

Appendix A – Jokes

I thought of doing a Appendectomy for this appendix but- what's a chapter on "Humor" without some jokes? I apologize in advance if:

> Any offend you;
> They're not funny;
> You've heard them before.

Also, I can't resist naming, and commenting on each joke:

1. Time and money—Everything is relative.
A man walking in the woods decided to ask God a question.
"God," the man said. "What is a million years to you?"
"What is a million years to you, is just a second to me."
"What is a million dollars to you?"
"What is a million dollars to you is just a penny to me."
"So God," the man said. "Can I have a penny?"
"Sure. Just a sec."

2. Watch what you say!
A man who smelled like a distillery flopped on a subway seat next to a priest. The man's tie was stained, his face was plastered with red lipstick, and a half empty bottle of gin was sticking out of his torn coat pocket. He opened his newspaper and began reading.
After a few minutes the disheveled guy turned to the priest and asked,
"Say, Father, what causes arthritis?"
"Mister, it's caused by loose living, being with cheap, wicked women, too much alcohol and a contempt for your fellow man."
"Well, I'll be damned!" the drunk muttered, returning to his paper.
The priest, thinking about what he had said, nudged the man and apologized.
"I'm very sorry. I didn't mean to come on so strong. How long have you had arthritis?"
"I don't have it, Father. I was just reading here that the Pope does."

3. How to get action!

A man looked out and saw that there were people in the shed stealing things.

He phoned the police, but they told him that no one was in his area to help, so he said ok, hung up, counted to 30, and phoned the police again.

"Hello. I just called you a few seconds ago because there were people in my shed.

Well, you don't have to worry about them now cause I've just shot them all."

Within five minutes there were half a dozen police cars in the area, an Armed Response unit, the works. Of course, they caught the burglars red-handed.

One of the policeman said to this man, "I thought you said that you'd shot them!"

He replied "I thought you said there was nobody available!"

4. Pronunciation *faux pas*
Man to attractive waitress:"How about a 'quickie'?"
Other man: "George – it's pronounced 'quiche'!"

Appendix B – Puzzles

One of the things that helped me recover from ARDS was rehabilitating my mind with puzzles which came from a variety of sources. Some of my favorites are:

1) You have 3 pills to take 1 every ½ hour: How long would it be before all the pills were taken?

2) Some months have 30 days and some months have 31 days. How many months have 28 days?

3) What do you get if you divide 30 by a half, and add 10?

4) A farmer had 17 sheep and all but 9 died. How many live sheep were left?

5) How many animals of each species did Moses take on the arc?

6) You are sleeping in a tent and get up at 7 a.m. and walk 1 mile south, then 1 mile east and 1 mile north, ending up back at your tent, where you shoot a bear. What color is the bear?

7) You have only one match and enter a cold dark room where there is an oil heater, an oil lamp and a candle. Which would you light first?

ANSWERS TO PUZZLES:

1) 1 hour

2) 12 (Every month has 28 days or more)

3) 70 (30 divided by 0.5 = 60 ...)

4) 9

5) It was Noah ...

6) White (polar bear at North Pole)

7) The match

MUSIC – A MAGICAL MEDICAL FORCE

"Music is the universal language of mankind."
Henry Wadsworth Longfellow

Life should begin and end with music. Music is analgesic for the woman delivering a baby, and soon after birth lullabies and other music are soothing to the newborn infant. Musical toys and music from any source have a calming affect on a growing child. Children, as they go through their teen-age years use music as a form of psychotherapy, even if some of the older generation find it hard to accept their choices. Adults in traffic jams may find music more soothing than news of daily disasters around the world. And finally, for the older person approaching death, music may bring back memories and provide a soothing influence for the anxious and/or depressed individual.

Throughout life music can be used to provide pain relief in dentistry, anxiety relief from a claustrophobic experience of MRIs, or a feeling of companionship for the hospitalized patient, whether alert or in a coma.

Music has long been used in tribal rituals and religious ceremonies (ancient and current) to evoke a physical as well as emotional response. An article by Don Campbell in the January-February 1998 issue of Natural Health notes that the Chinese produce music for specific ailments, including obesity and constipation! The Chinese and Japanese prescribe music as they would an herbal medicine. He notes the roots of music reach back to the dawn of civilization and suggests the possibility that dance and song preceded speech.

Campbell observes that many different kinds of music can be therapeutic, according to the particular individual. He notes, however, the "Mozart Effect" … the special ability of Mozart's music to heal a wide cross-section of ailments. More than any other music, the sounds of Mozart surpass all others in studies of the healing effect of music, as shown by Alfred Tomatis, M.D., a French physician, who has spent his professional career studying the healing powers of music, the Mozart Effect in particular.

Hilding H. Olson published an article in July 1999 issue of the

King County Medical Society Bulletin, "Music, Medicine and Surgery", in which he notes the historic inter-dependence of music and medicine. Dr. Theodore Billroth (1827-1894) was both a musician and a surgeon and a close associate of Johannes Brahms (1833-1897). To this day there is a high correlation of musical and medical interest. In my case, I must confess that I dropped out of piano lessons in grade school. I participated in a triple quartet, the "Zumbyes", while at Amhurst College and I still bring music to my patients as I sing some song when entering the clinic exam room ... "sing ... sing a song ..."

Music, accompanying exercise, may be a stimulant to aerobic and muscle building exercises, which are beneficial to health and physical rehabilitation. One's aerobic capacity seems greater when listening to music.

One's "spiritual capacity" is elevated by music which is such a prominent part of many church services. I am still excited by the sound and reverberations of a church organ. Music and words together have a particularly powerful impact.

In my own case, I am told that music was played in my room much of the day while I was in a coma. My family knows I love music and chose the types of music I like best. (I don't know if they knew about the Mozart Effect, but I recovered, in any case). On my birthday, February 2nd, five days following my January 28th accident, my family sang the familiar "Happy Birthday" song and I am told that a tear came to my eye while I was unconscious.

Later, in my rehabilitation phase, I chose tapes of music that made the time and pain pass more easily. Still later, after I went home, but was still too weak to get out and about, I used music to help me regain my sense of wellness. Instead of a funeral, we held a "Celebration of Life Party", featuring the "Ain't No Heaven Seven" Jazz Band, a group of physicians including two of my friends, Terry Rogers and Ward Kennedy. It was their CD that buoyed my spirits while hospitalized. About a hundred others were lifted by the jazz performance and my evident recovery (I was looking at the grass from the green down instead of from the roots up).

I learned of Greg Fleckenstein in Michigan. Greg is a recovered ARDS patient who has over 5,000 albums of music in his personal collection. He has been willing to make two tapes for any individual who wants to use music for therapy. The patient can choose the exact selections or simply specify the type of music he or she likes. In my case, I chose Dixieland Jazz for one tape, and up-beat gospel music (none of the "woe-is-me I'm a sinner" type). I used these tapes for many months of my early recovery. Greg's can email address is: cgf2722@novagate.com., Muskegon Music Ministries, 1423 Moody Street, Whitehall, MI 49461 Greg's own ARDS experience is related in the section of this book on Inspirational Stories.

Another Inspirational Story is told in this book by Shannon Kalisher, who was helped by Willow, a Music Therapist, who put Shannon's words to music. Be sure to read Shannon's story!

Music is used in general hospitals to elevate mood and promote relaxation of patients. In my limited experience, I have not witnessed formal music therapy, but I personally benefited from the musical tapes provided by Greg Fleckenstein and my family. In that regard, I encourage families to bring in favorite music for their loved one who is a patient, even if in a coma.

The internet provides a number of references where music is used for therapy in chronic medical conditions. The American Lung Association has an interest in ARDS and is working with a group of us organizing national conferences on ARDS. Music therapy is an important element of healing discussed in these conferences. Check out website: www.nwards.org.

Music therapy is actually much more professionalized than I realized. From an internet search I learned about The American Music Therapy Association formed in 1998 as a union of two other associations (AMTA 8455 Colesville Road, Suite 1000, Silver Spring, Maryland 20910, phone 301-589-3300). I learned that the first music therapy degree program was founded at Michigan State University in 1944.

SUMMARY

In an era of computers and high technology medicine, it is essential to remember music as an important element of healing beyond medicine.

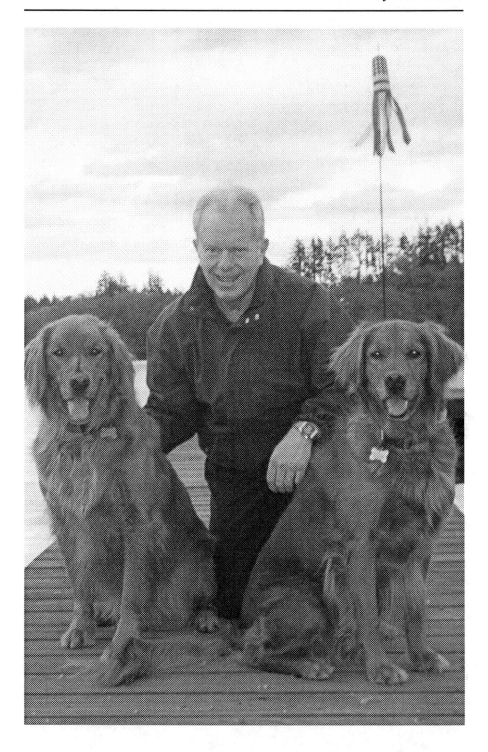

PETS
PERFECT PROVIDERS FOR HEALTH & HEALING

"Throughout history animals have played a significant role in human customs, legends, and religions. Primitive people found that human-animal relationships were important to their very survival, and pet-keeping was common in hunter-gatherer societies. In our own time, the great increase in pet ownership may reflect a largely urban population's often unsatisfied need for intimacy, nurture, and contact with nature".

National Institutes of Health (NIH) Workshop, 1987 (Ref. 1)

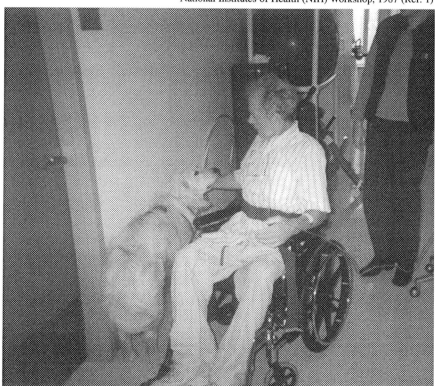

Pet Therapy with "Rainier"
at Harborview Rehab Center.

Sandy, an 18-year-old student was near death with ARDS in the ICU until her family snuck in her pet puppy, "Mitzi", with the message that Mitzi missed her and wanted her to come home. A doggie kiss on the cheek sealed the deal and within a few hours Sandy's condition improved, eventually leading to a return to home - and to Mitzi.

Proof of "Pet Power?"- - No. But a better outcome than predicted with the best that medical care had to offer prior to Mitzi.

My own recovery from ARDS was helped by "Rainier", a Golden Retriever on the Rehab Floor at Harborview Hospital. With Rainier's encouragement I progressed from wheelchair to walker and increased the length of my walks. And, with my peripheral neuropathy (tingling of my finger tips) I enjoyed petting Rainier and practicing my puppy patter. But would my own Golden Retriever, "Cinco de Mayo," be jealous? If so, it didn't show on my day passes when Cinco's doggie delight was so evident on our reunions. On my discharge to home after a total of 92 hospital days it was all love, licks, bounding, and tail-wagging joy from Cinco.

In my outpatient Rehab, Cinco was a patient coach as my walking improved from use of a walker to a cane to unassisted walking for longer and longer distances (though now measured in yards instead of miles, pre-ARDS). During the long hours alone, I always had a companion, always loving, never critical, never negative. No wonder I had such a positive outlook and rapid recovery! Pet power!!

More than half of all U.S. households have one or more pets. Pets are more common in households with children, yet there are more pets than children in American households. There are more than 51 million dogs, 56 million cats, 45 million birds, 75 million small mammals and reptiles, and uncounted millions of aquarium fish, according to a working group from the National Institutes of Health (NIH) Workshop, 1987 (Ref. 1).

Since ancient times, Man has had animals as companions and healers. Rennie (Ref. 2) notes that the ancient Greeks believed dogs could cure ailments and kept them as co-therapists in their healing temples. Aescalapius, the Greek God of Healing, used "sacred dogs" in his healing temples.

"The use of horseback riding for people with serious disabilities has been reported for centuries. In 1792, animals were incorporated into the treatment for mental patients at the York Retreat, England, as part of an enlightened approach attempting to reduce the use of harsh drugs and restraints. The first suggested use of animals in a therapeutic setting in the United States was in 1919 at St. Elizabeth's Hospital in Washington, D. C., when Superintendent Dr. W.A. White received a letter from Secretary of the Interior F.K. Lane suggesting the use of dogs as companions for the psychiatric hospital's resident patients. Following this, the earliest extensive use of companion animals in the United States occurred from 1944 to 1945 at an Army Air Corps Convalescent Hospital at Pawling, New York. Patients recovering from war experiences were encouraged to work at the hospital's farm with hogs, cattle, horses, and poultry. After the war, modest efforts began in using animals in outpatient psychotherapy. During the 1970s, numerous case studies of animals facilitating therapy with children and senior citizens were reported." (Ref. 1)

Since psychological factors are important in cardiovascular disease, it seems reasonable that pets would provide a positive influence. The coronary-prone behavior pattern (Type A behavior) of anger and time-pressured living may well be modified through association with pets. Stress management is known to reduce blood pressure. Pets precede pharmacology to provide stress management.

Few evidence-based reports on pet therapy are available. Results from one study (Ref. 1) indicate that post-myocardial infarction (heart attack) survival rates are higher among pet owners than among non-owners. It is possible that myocardial infarction (MI) patients who are pet owners are in better health, and therefore able to take care of household pets.

Although most of us have pets, and humans have a long history of association with animals, it is only recently that the health benefits of this human-animal bonding have been recognized and studied. Dr. Sandra Barker, in Virginia, has numerous publications on this topic, including an excellent review in the February 1999 issue of *Psychiatric Times*. (Ref. 18) She notes the early (1980) report of Friedman (Ref. 3) that pet owners had a significantly higher one-year survival from a myocardial infarction than did non-pet owners. Approximately 6% of pet owners versus 28% of non-pet owners died within one year after hospitalization. Pet ownership was associated with increased survival independent of severity of disease and for non-dog pet owners as well (cat-owners, etc.).

A 1992 report from Australia by Anderson (Ref. 5) showed pet owners had lower blood pressure and triglyceride levels than did their counterparts. Barker (Ref. 18) gives other references which allege:

❖ a decrease in minor health ailments in pet owners
❖ lower utilization of physician services among pet-owning
❖ Medicare recipients experiencing stressful life events
❖ less stress in medical procedures when a dog is present

AAT (Animal-Assisted Therapy) traces back to "Hippotherapy" (therapeutic horseback riding) in the 18th century. Riding was used to improve balance, posture, coordination and joint function. Horseback riding improves the mood of patients needing crutches or wheelchairs.

A study by Serpell in 1991 reported dog owners had increased walking and self-esteem as possible mechanisms for the health benefits of dog ownership. (Ref. 4) This study and others are well discussed in the book "The Waltham Book of Human-Animal Interactions: Benefits and Responsibilities".

Not all aspects of pet ownership are necessarily positive. Barking dogs and meowing cats may be a source of irritation. Pet care can be costly. Dog messes are annoying. I like the joke – "I wondered whether to get a puppy or a wife. I couldn't decide whether to ruin my carpet or my life." All said and done, there would appear to be more health benefits than hazards in pet ownership.

The mechanism for health benefits associated with pets is not entirely clear. It seems likely that the unconditional love of a pet would be beneficial. Reduction of anxiety and depression associated with pet companionship may be a central benefit. Pets also give their owners a sense of purpose and responsibility – a reason to live. People who walk their dogs may be said to be "walked by their dog" to the health benefits of each.

Although studies are important, individual stories are often more moving. Bill Cole writes me about how his dog "Ted" was not only his friend and caretaker, but had a story of his own. Any of us going through angioplasty and clinical depression would be glad to have a dog like "Ted." This is a story where Dog and Man care for each other in times of need.

Ted the Lhasa, helped me recover from emergency heart angioplasty and subsequent major vascular surgery, while I was also clinically depressed. His contribution was spiritual, and also as an example to me of how he plowed through his own physical hardships. Sometimes he would get me to sit with him on the back porch, where it seemed like he was telling me stories about his long and gallant service.

Remember the time I tried to chase off the German Shepherd and he chased me all the way from the front yard to under our own dining table? I don't scare easily, but that was one time. Remember that god awful Japanese dog that wanted to tear out my throat. I must have muttered something about his mother, and he understood Tibetan...Remember how long I was in the hospital after I was wounded? And you guys visited me twice a day? And you made me a pen when I got home, that you scooted around the living room so I could have sunshine?

Ted had been tumbled by two cars, badly fracturing his hip and a lot of other things. He was a trooper about all the treatment and recovery, and never complained about his limp or cold days. Ted didn't have a grumbly bone in his body unless it required dogly defensive action against intruder dogs. In spite of his own problems, Ted was always at my side caring for me.

About 50 stories of remarkable actions of animals in warning, rescuing or helping the healing process in their human partners are told in **"Animal Miracles-Inspirational and Heroic True Stories"** by Brad and Sherry Steiger, published in 1999 (Ref. 7). General health benefits are summarized showing that pets can:

- ❖ Lower blood pressure
- ❖ Cut cholesterol
- ❖ Minimize stress
- ❖ Lessen pain perception
- ❖ Decrease loneliness and depression
- ❖ Reduce breakups of marriage
- ❖ Increase longevity
- ❖ Predict seizures

In another story told to me, Jeanie Knecht tells about how her dogs, C.J. and Kelsie, helped her recover from ARDS when she was expected to die.

> *My family told me that all the doctors said I was going to die and they made me a DNR. Everybody was saying various things to try and get me to respond, but I never moved a muscle. When it finally looked hopeless, my sister said to me, "C.J. and Kelsie are fine. They are waiting for you." She said I squeezed her hand and everybody in the room, including the nurses started crying. My sister said she knew then that I was going to make it.*
>
> *My two dogs were the motivation to get me back home and recovering. I don't think I would have fought to live so hard if I didn't have them.*

In "**Dogs Never Lie About Love**", (Ref. 8), Jeffrey Masson presents a masterful analysis of the emotional world of dogs and their relations with humans, including the love and loyalty of dogs for their human partners. Masson is aware that "anecdotal data" (stories) differ from controlled laboratory-type studies but both types of information may improve our understanding of our world. Reliable observations on specific experiences - even "miracles" or "exceptions from the rule" may, in fact lead to paradigm shifts - i.e. new models of thought. I believe that analysis of stories of the healing power of pets may lead us to a greater understanding of healing itself.

More stories about pets as teachers and healers are presented in "Chicken Soup for the Pet Lover's Soul" by Jack Canfield, with Mark Victor Hansen, Marty Becker and Carol Kline, published in 1998. The authors note, "There are many stories about a pet's power to comfort and even to heal. Our pets keep us from getting sick as often, and if we do become sick, we recover faster. Taken together, the evidence is overwhelming: Pets are good for our hearts, bodies and souls."

Here are two stories sent to me giving case-specific evidence of the healing power of pets in ARDS.

Heather Favale: *"I am a 31-year old health education teacher who had ARDS two years ago. I was in a coma for four weeks and was given a 10% chance of survival. A priest was called in to read me my last rites. With lots of love, prayer, and God, I pulled through. I was told I would never run again. But keeping up with my ten pets (6 cats and 4 dogs), helped train me to the point where one year after my release from the hospital, I completed a mini-triathlon.*"

Linda Silva: "*My dog Gizmo came to see me in the rehabilitation hospital. I was worried he wouldn't remember me. After all, he hadn't seen me in two months. When my mother brought him in to visit me for the first time, I remember being so overjoyed. He actually tried to jump on my lap in the wheelchair. When I went home, I could barely walk, but Gizmo patiently helped me with my rehabilitation until I could walk again.*"

As shown in Eric Gebelein's story (Ref. 9), pets have a true value as companions in health and illness. In an article, "**The Therapeutic Use of Companion Animals**" (Ref. 10) it is stated that, "there is increasing evidence that pets not only improve 'quality of life', but can also improve measurable 'quantity of life'. For example, research studies have reported marked reduction in risk factors for cardiovascular disease in groups of pet owners compared with non-owners. In another study, pet owners had significantly lower serum triglyceride levels, compared with non-pet owners. The authors give seven Internet resources for pet therapy which are listed in the Reference section at the end of the chapter.

There appears to be some unexplained powers of animals which are not yet explained.

Deb Rebel's story told to me:

"Our four-legged therapist cat is the master of "purr therapy". He is the best gauge of whether you are really sick or not. You crawl into bed to die from whatever it is, and if he comes and parks near you, unbidden, to gently lie touching you and gently purring, comfortingly-- you're ill."

The ability of a homing pigeon to find "home" when released miles away has been well studied but not yet understood. The ability of dogs to smell and to hear high-pitch sounds are incredible skills which are understood but many other skills are not. Rupert Sheldrake published "<u>Dogs That Know When Their Owners Are Coming Home -</u>

And Other Unexplained Powers Of Animals" in 1999 (Three Rivers Press, Random House, NYC). This is an incredible book which deals profoundly with questions of animal powers and the human mind. For example, he relates experimental studies confirming the human power of feeling when we are being stared at. Details are given in his website at www.sheldrake.org.

Sheldrake attributes the healing power of dogs and cats to the unconditional love they give. And he notes, even Sigmund Freud was assisted by his dog with the "petting cure".

Animal Assisted Therapy Programs

Doctors have been slow to accept what countless individuals have experienced with pets as elements of healing. The medical establishment is coming around however. Harborview Hospital in Seattle has an Animal Assisted Therapy Program using dogs to enhance rehabilitation and healing. When I was in Harborview, on the Rehabilitation Ward, my spirits were buoyed by "Rainier" as I discussed at the beginning of this chapter. The Spring 2001 Harborview Viewpoint describes how "Archer", a black Labrador mix, helps patients regain hand coordination by being groomed. Others work on speech therapy, giving Archer verbal commands. Both Archer and Rainier are part of the Canine Companion Program (www.caninecompanions.org).

The Delta Foundation was established in 1977 in Portland, Oregon, under the leadership of Michael McCulloch, MD. Delta's founders wanted to understand the quality of the relationship between pet owners, pets, and care givers, both human and veterinary. Delta's early years focused on funding the first credible research on why animals are important to the general population and specifically how they affect health and well being. Once the importance of animals in everyday lives was established from this research, Delta began to look at how animals can change the lives of people who are ill and disabled. In the late 1980s, Delta began creating educational materials to apply the scientific information in everyday life. Membership expanded to pet owners and a broader general public.

In the 1990's, Delta built on its scientific and educational base to provide direct services at the local level. This includes providing the first comprehensive training in animal-assisted activities and therapy to volunteers and health care professionals. A significant advance was the development of the *Standards of Practice in Animal-Assisted Activities and Animal-Assisted Therapy*, which provides guidance in the administrative structure of AAA/T programs, including animal selection, personnel training, treatment plan development, documentation and more. Use of the *Standards of Practice in Animal-Assisted Activities and Animal-Assisted Therapy* provides a sound base on which to build quality AAA/T programs. (Ref. 13)

One of the most impressive programs is Rx: DOG LOVE, Inc., founded in 1991 in Akron, Ohio under the auspices of the Delta Society. It was founded by Bonnie Dillon, C.E.N., who was Head Nurse in the Emergency Department at Akron City. Handlers and pets are licensed jointly to operate in health facilities in northeastern Ohio. It served as a model for many hospital based programs across the country and overseas. Rx: Dog Love serves hospital patients and educates the community about the benefits of animals in health care.

The 2002 President of Rx: DOG LOVE, Inc., Beth Fink, contributes the following description:

> *We value what we do and we are humbled by it. The powerful connection that an animal can make to a human in distress, in pain, in grief, in confusion, is valid and is documentable. While the formal terminology, "Animal-assisted Activity and Animal-assisted Therapy" are fairly recent, the concept dates back to the 16th century. Even in those medically primitive times, animals were found to calm and sooth psychiatric patients. Florence Nightingale stressed the importance of a little singing bird to brighten the mood (brightened affect) of a hospitalized patient. So, it's not new what we do! There are numerous research studies and articles as proof.....measurable and documented.*
>
> *The success we and many other programs of AAA/AAT have had is due in large part to the selection of suitable, appropriate animals and handlers. Delta Society is the nation's foremost registry of suitable animals and handlers for work as volunteers in prisons, rehab centers, acute care settings, assisted living centers, schools, Alzheimer Care Centers, long term care facilities, psychiatric facilities, etc.*

Delta, founded in 1977, evaluates both ends of the leash...handler, too, for suitability! Then, they require training of the handler to familiarize them with working with different patient populations, recognizing stress in the patient/client, the animal, and themselves, Infection Control, liability matters, proper presentation, safety etc.

The animal (dogs, cats, horses, ponies, guinea pigs, hamsters, certain parrots, pot bellied pigs, goats, rabbits are all eligible for evaluation and registration as Delta Society Pet Partners!) undergoes an evaluation for skills and aptitude, as does the handler. The animal undergoes a health screening by a veterinarian, in more detail than the usual once a year pet-to-the-vet exam! Then, annually, the animal must be re-screened for health suitability, and every two years, there is a reassessment of skills and aptitude of both handler and animal.

In Akron, the Prescription: DOG LOVE program was the first AAA/AAT program in an adult acute care setting in Northern Ohio! We began in 1991. We continue to participate in research studies, in therapy projects, and serve the hospitalized patient, the facility and staff with nearly 2000 hours a year of volunteer service.

Beth continues:

We have been with patients at the moment of death. We have been used as a treatment modality upon physician order in the Intensive Care Unit. We have been used to relieve stress in staff and patient, alike. In this day of modern medicine, while technological advances are developed at breathtaking speed, the wise physician understands, but perhaps cannot explain, the power of the human-animal bond. Among the monitors, blinking lights, digital read outs, state of the art machinery, there is, in more and more critical care arenas, a "healer" that does not come wrapped in sterile stainless steel......but rather in a clean soft fur coat with no agenda other than to offer unconditional love. I LOVE what I do! I am grateful to God for the opportunity to do what I do....and it's so simple. It's so natural, and non-threatening. The animal accepts the patient at his level of wellness, regardless of his state of mind or body, regardless of his station in life. And isn't this the key? The human knows the animal's generosity; the human knows that the animal offers unconditional love, unconditional acceptance.

Beth Fink provides five case examples involving AAA/AAT at Summa Health System, Akron, Ohio, and at Akron general Medical Center, Akron, Ohio:

Case #1: Patient Weaned From Vent.

Elderly gentleman in our ICU (Akron City Hospital) on a trach. Despondent. When nurses would start weaning parameters, the patient would panic and have anxiety attacks, preventing him from being weaned.

Every day, on physician order, an animal-handler team would visit this patient in the ICU. The volunteer would drape the patient's bed linen with a clean sheet and place the dog on the bed beside the patient. The volunteer would talk to the man about the program and about the dog, and would ask "yes and no" questions of the man. As he stroked and patted the dog and visited with the volunteer, nurse observed his level of anxiety lessened and could decrease the vent setting. After 7 days of visits with the animal-handler team, patient was completely weaned from the vent and was able to be sent to a nursing home for skilled intensive rehab.

Case #2: Post-Extubation Care

Young man had been admitted to ICU (Akron City Hospital) and had been unresponsive secondary to acute infection. The day the patient was extubated (after 30 days), the animal-handler team visited the patient. He looked at the dog, then at his nurses, and nodded vigorously, indicating that he was eager to visit with the dog. Clean linen was placed on the bed, and the dog was lifted onto the bed beside the patient.

His hands were taken out of restraints and he began to stroke the dog with both hands. He fully extended both his arms to touch the dog, and stroked the dog's ears and face using his fingertips, flexing his fingers and wrists. The Physical Therapist was at bedside and joked with the patient, "Well, I guess you don't need me here!"

The patient reached up and moved his mask aside and said "When is the last time someone fed this dog?" (making reference to the fact that the English Springer Spaniel, Nathan, in the bed was "well-rounded")

The Rx: DOG LOVE teams followed this patient daily on physician order throughout his entire hospital stay, during his intensive care stay, through the rehab unit, and until he was released from the hospital.

Case #3: "Best Medicine Yet"

Elderly female patient, at Akron General Medical Center was alert and oriented. Despondent. Had a dog at home which was being cared for by her family. Several health related incidents had delayed her release from the hospital for over 3 weeks. Nurses requested daily dog visits to this patient. After having been visited by several of the animal-handler teams, the patient said to her nurse that this was the best medicine she ever had and she was going to get better because her little dog needed her at home.

Her depression lessened, she began to eat her meals, and she was eventually released to her residence with assistance.

Case #4: Dog Love in Unresponsive Patient

Young man, age 16, motor vehicle accident in ICU at Akron City Hospital. Traumatic brain injury. Unresponsive. With nursing staff watching, Animal-handler team visited this young man, placed his hands on the dog's head, stuffed the dog's furry ear inside patient's clenched hand. Volunteer described each thing she was doing with the dog, described the dog, the breed and color, talked about the program. After ten minutes, the volunteer looked up at the door to this patient's room. The Intensivist had observed this patient's monitors throughout the dog's visit from the nurses' station in the center of the unit and then came to the patient's room to observe the interaction. He instructed the nurses and the volunteer present that he was ordering daily visits from the teams for this young man. The Rx: DOG LOVE teams followed this patient throughout his hospital stay. They participated in "increased stimulation" and daily physical therapy sessions with the therapist. After two weeks in ICU, the patient would follow commands re: reaching for the dog's ear or foot. He would follow the dog with his eyes as the dog entered or left the room. Nursing and/PT had not been able to get these responses from this patient. Patient ultimately was discharged to a rehab facility.

Case #5: End Stage Cancer Terminal Care

45-Year Old female patient in Oncology unit, on Comfort Care. End stage cancer, on trach. Teams made several visits to this patient over 8 days. On the last day of life, the physician asked the team to visit this patient. Family was in the room waiting for the death. Clean linen was placed on the patient's bed and the dog was placed beside the patient. The patient was non-responsive. Volunteer spoke to the patient as if she were awake, and that she was the dog's favorite person to visit. The patient's hands were placed on the dog's head and ears and stroked over the dog, just as before. The volunteer told her how much the dog enjoyed visiting with her. When the dog was removed from the bed and the linen was rolled and disposed of, the family thanked the volunteer profusely for the visits to their family member. They told the volunteer that this experience was made easier because of the visit and the softened memory that they would take with them of the death experience.

These are five impressive cases showing the impact of DOG LOVE teams in ICU patients. In cases like these, stories speak louder than statistics. For those interested in more descriptive reports, see the websites of "Pawprints and Purrs" and "Dog-Play.com".

Pawprints and Purrs (www.sniksnak.com) is an extensive website, including information on pet therapy examples for all ages and many clinical conditions, including the following:

- ❖ Attention Deficit Disorder (ADD)
- ❖ Depression
- ❖ Anxiety
- ❖ Alzheimer's
- ❖ Touch-Deprived

Diane Blackman has a wonderful website, www.dog-play.com, that provides extensive information related to pet therapy and other topics. She notes that visiting with animals can help people feel less lonely, and less depressed. Visits from dogs can provide a welcome change from routine, or the renewal of old friendships. People become more active and responsive both during and after visiting with animals.

An animal visit can offer entertainment or a welcome distraction from pain and infirmity. People often talk to the dogs, and share with them their thoughts and feelings and memories. Animal visits provide something to look forward to. Stroking a dog or cat can reduce a person's blood pressure. Petting encourages use of hands and arms, stretching and turning.

Blackman believes that a pet makes it easier for two strangers to talk. It gives people a common interest and provides a focus for conversation. Many people in hospitals or group homes have had to give up pet ownership and they miss the casual acceptance a pet gives them. A dog pays little attention to age or physical ability, but accepts people as they are. The benefits continue even after the visit. The visit leaves behind memories not only of the visit, but of past experiences. It offers something for people to share.

A national directory of Animal Assisted Therapy Programs can be found at www.activitytherapy.com/us.htm.

<u>SUMMARY</u>

I propose that we recognize pets as one of the most perfect providers of health care from prevention to treatment to rehabilitation to the days leading to death itself. Whether imaginary, stuffed-toy or any of a variety of living animals, PETS are important contributors to health and healing. My own healing recovery from ARDS was helped by "Rainier" a companion Golden Retriever in Harborview Hospital. And when I came home to continue rehabilitation, I had at my side our Golden Retriever, Cinco. She exuded happiness and love and reminded me to play and to sleep and appreciate the meaning of each day one at a time.

Appendix A: Personal History With Pets

Pets are an Element of Healing for both psychological and physical problems. I will discuss my own experiences with pets to show their importance in my life.

Dogs - Love & Loss Lessons

My ARDS experiences with pets were not the first which convinced me about "Pet Power." Growing up in Iowa, Ohio and Michigan, my family always had a dog - except for those painful periods following the death of one of these special members of our family. This experience of loss by death, and re-establishment of life after grief is one of the main lessons in pet-people relationships. (I prefer not to call it pet Ownership.) As an element of healing, pets prepare us for facing death - that of loved ones and that of ourselves. We learn how to handle loss of a loved one through tears and time. Though never replacing the lost loved one (pet, person or part of ourselves), we learn to *move on* and to find joy again in life. We know that adding a pet can restore meaning and love in a life that is lonely and suffering loss.

My experiences with laughter and play with puppies and kittens, as they mature to dogs and cats, also have been healing, particularly in times of stress or boredom. And I've learned that playfulness can continue in maturity!

Dog friends have been - and are - important elements of healing and happiness in my life, but there are other animal friends that have been part of my life. As I cared for these pets, they cared for me. Some of these pet stories, like the next one, are rather unusual and amusing.

Rat Responses

Pet animals can create health-promoting laughter and surprise in others as well as ourselves. While I was in a biology class at Amherst College, I spared the life of a white rat that was used in some experiments on semi-synthetic diets. I'd become quite attached to "Heavy" whom I raised from a baby to a heavy adult and I couldn't bear the thought of me being a rat and "sacrificing" him. So, Heavy got his own caged room in mine. Being tame-to-touch and easy to carry,

Heavy often went out with me as a passenger in my front sport coat pocket where he traveled comfortably with his nose and eyes just peeking out. I must admit he looked cute and was quite a hit in my tuxedo at the prom! Even rats can be tamed - and fun! And who would have thought that a rat could be an element of happiness and healing?

Turtle Pets

While I'm sharing pet parables, each with its own significance as an element of healing, I must tell the story of "Fang", my pet turtle in high school days in Hudson, Ohio. I found Fang when each of us was walking through the woods. He begged me, and later taught me, to *slow down!* He agreed (in turtle-talk) to come live with me in my room. Fang was also a pocket pal and helped me learn to slow down and to pull back my head if in danger (too bad I couldn't do that when I fell off the ski lift!). The next time you are troubled, think of a turtle as a terrific, tame pet that can go where other pets are not allowed. It will not set off metal detectors but may be found if you're frisked. It makes a perfect gift for the person who has nothing - or everything! Sadly, turtles tend to wander off as Fang did over 50 years ago, but turtles live a long time so maybe there's still hope that we'll meet again. If so, he'll be pleased to note how I've slowed down! By the way, Fang is pronounced with a resonant lisp as a prolonged sound. Pfffaaaaannnghhhh!…a name that Jerry Florez and I created to cause laughter for no other reason than how we said it. So, for a low-maintenance pet to remind you to slow down, think "turtle". It may also remind you to pull back in your shell and keep quiet at certain times of danger, when your health is in danger!

Charles the Cat

Over the years I've had several cats but none so memorable as "Charles" - because he WAS a Charles! Charles appeared at my doorstep one day when I was still a bachelor and made me a deal too good to refuse: "I'll keep the rats, dogs and burglars away if you'll feed me and take me in at night."……"Sounds good to me, you feline fox, you," I said, "but don't forget the mice, birds and raccoons!" …"Yeah, I lost this ear wrestling with a raccoon," Charles meowed, whistfully. So, Charles and I hit it off like long-lost soul mates and, I must say, Charles was a hit with my children and all those who visited us.

Charles taught us that Love and Independence go together, as other cat lovers have learned. Sadly, one day Charles simply didn't show up for work, play, food or love. There's still a tear in my eye as I think about Charles, hoping he found a better place though suspecting he fell victim to the "Laws of Nature"(Who says they are laws?) and satisfied the raccoon for whom an ear was not enough. As I wipe away the moisture from my eye I realize that, once again, a pet has been a teacher and an element of healing. Charles taught me that I must move on from the loss of love of a very special being. His Spirit lives on within me. Perhaps he and Fang have met somewhere, as they have within me.

Fish

This is a "fish story" which is almost true. It is true that fish can get to know you and provide interest and pet-power for health and healing. Folks should fathom a fish tank if they can't have a dog or cat or other furry critter, due to allergies or apartment/condo living restrictions,. Watching those shiny, colorful, speedy swimmers can provide hours of delight and distraction. It may sound fishy but an aquarium can be good for your health, as it was in my case. Here's the story:

Lynn and I had had a 45-gallon aquarium for several years and in the home phase of my recuperation from ARDS I enjoyed watching these colorful creatures flashing back and forth in choreographic splendor. "Hard to believe we evolved from them," I thought. But I felt a healing sense of nature as I watched them and thought, "If a fish were to get ARDS it would be all over…fini….caput…done!"

Gradually, with or without ARDS, our original mixed school of tropical fish dwindled to two grey something-or-others. Without telling our kids, we decided to let nature take its course and when these two survivors were gone we would replace the gravel and start with a new class of colored fish. But - our plans never floated since our thoughtful children decided, while we were out-of-town, to add two young fish to the tank. These tiny two fish, each under an inch in length, were hard to find in our 45-gallon tank. But not for long! Within a month they doubled in size and did so again the next month - to our great delight until they ate the original two fish. "Perhaps that was a 'natural death' after all," we rationalized. But, after two more doublings the larger of the two new fish ate the other. That left one, still-growing fish whose name, in deference to his size, was "Hugo"(pronounced Huge - O).

With no competition Hugo continued to grow till he nearly filled the 45-gallon tank. With our love of animals and our desire to make Hugo happy, we purchased a 75-gallon home for Hugo, moving him into his new habitat with a large gauze sling. Hugo is now bigger by far than the average fisherman's catch - even bigger than "the one that got away."

Hugo lives on, and is HUGE - though I may have exaggerated a few facts for the sake of a better "fish story." But the fact is a fish tank can be a calming and useful element of healing in a hospital room, doctor's office or patient's home or nursing home.

"Dog Tales for the Heart"

This is the name of a wonderful little book, subtitled "Stories of Hope, Love and Wisdom", edited by Sue Hershkowitz, a "CSP"(Certified Speaking Professional) of the NSA (National Speakers Association). I am proud to be a member of NSA and to have a story, "The Nature of Love", in her book. Published in 1995 by High Impact Publications, in Scotsdale, AZ 85254 (Phone 602 996 8864- have fun and give her a call!)

The "Dog Tale" I tell relates to our, now deceased, Golden Retriever, "Melekalikimaka," ("Mele"), who we trained to love and protect four baby ducks which were being attacked by crows. As the ducklings grew they imprinted on Mele and slept with her and followed her in daily walks around the yard. By the end of summer the ducks were large enough to fly away and swim away - which they did! I concluded, "Love is learned. That's the way it works in nature!" If ducks can be helped by "Dog love", how much more can humans be helped?

Bunny Buddies

Another animal healer was "Reno", the rabbit. Reno and Mele also learned to get along and play chase with each other. When Lynn and I found that we were too busy to give Reno the attention she deserved, we gave her away to some friends with a young child. This seemed like giving up a child for adoption! At least we didn't say, "Hare today-Gone Tomorrow!" How do hares help healing? Darned if I know!

Horsing Around

I am convinced that horses help healing. They're not exactly lap-pets or bed partners however! Nevertheless a horse can give and receive love - which is a healing element. Also, horseback riding isn't exactly stage 1 of physical rehabilitation after a long hospitalization. Riding, however, is a goal which motivates exercise and therefore is part of the healing process.

In my case, I've done more horsing around than horseback riding but I do have a childhood story with some learning experiences from a ride alone on a horse when I was six years old. This story has been published in a heart-warming collection of essays called "GRAND-STORIES - 101+BRIDGES of LOVE JOINING GRANDPARENTS and GRANDKIDS", compiled and edited by Ernie Wendell, and published in 2000 by *Friendly Oaks Publications*, P.O. Box 662, Pleasanton, TX 78064. (Phone 830-569-3586)

My contribution to this book tells the story of my visit with "Bompy", my maternal grandfather, at his summer cabin in the backwoods of Iowa. As a 6-year old I had little horse-riding experience but persuaded Bompy to let me ride his horse. "O.K., but if you get lost just let go of the reins and the horse will bring you home!", Bompy advised. As described in Wendell's book, I did get lost and was brought back home when I let go of the reins. There were several "learning experiences" from this experience. The most general lesson is the metaphor that reminds us that in life there are times to let go of the reins - and be shown the way home. Horses have many lessons to teach (as do grandfathers) and have a special kind of loving, healing relationship with us humans.

Stuffed and Story Pets -Imaginary Animals

I can make the point that every bed-ridden person should have the option of having a stuffed animal to promote health and healing. Cuddling with, and talking to, a stuffed animal bed-partner, which talks back in your imagination, just has to be good for your health - mentally and physically!

As a child I was protected by my two teddy bears who played with me during the day and slept with me at night. Recently I learned where the name "Teddy Bear" originated. Teddy refers to Theodore ("Teddy") Roosevelt who, on a hunting trip in the early 1900's, spared the life of a mother bear with its cub. The media, charmed by this tender act, published a raft of cartoons showing Teddy with a bear, which soon was drawn as a cub. When an English manufacturer of stuffed animals sent a shipment of stuffed toy bear cubs to the U.S.A., they were promptly dubbed "Teddy Bears"! (Ref: *Alex Stevens, MD, review of book "Theodore Rex", reviewed in May, 2002 issue of King County Med. Soc. Bul)*

Walt Disney deserves the credit for developing Mickey Mouse, Donald Duck and the whole yardful of talking animals that have played into our hearts for the past century.

Puff "The Magic Dragon" and fictional heroes such as "Lassie" have captured our imagination giving us humor and hope, whatever our condition might be.

We learn to love and relate to stuffed animals, toy animals and book-character animals within the first few months of life and throughout childhood. Why stop? It's not healthy to feel lonely. With a stuffed animal, and a good imagination, you are never alone! And, if you are wondering what to GIVE to a Patient - - this is it!......A stuffed animal!

Summary

I attribute much of my health and happiness to the pets that have been part of my life from birth to the present. I have related some of the stories without "proving" the health-power of these real, toy and imaginary companions. Yet I know that the unconditional love of my dogs, in particular, has been a major element in my stability in sickness, stress and sadness.

Appendix B: Humor and Pets

I.

A dog who has been shot in the front foot walks into a bar with his foot bandaged and says, "...I'm looking for the man who shot my paw!"

II.

If you can start the day without caffeine or pep pills,
If you can be cheerful, ignoring aches and pains,
If you can resist complaining and boring people with your troubles,
If you can eat the same food everyday and be grateful for it,
If you can conquer tension without liquor or pills,
If you can sleep without the aid of drugs,
If you can do all these things...

THEN YOU ARE PROBABLY THE FAMILY DOG

III.

"Plus je vois les hommes, plus j'admire les chiens"
Madame Roland, 18th Century
(The more I see men, the more I admire dogs)
or
The more I get to know men, the more I like my dog!

<u>REFERENCES</u>

National Institutes of Health (NIH) Workshop, 1987
    www.woofs.org/psychology/petstudy/omar1.html

Rennie, "The Therapeutic Relationship between Animals and Humans," Society for Companion Animal Studies Journal, 9:4, 1997.

Friedmann, E., Katcher, A. H., Lynch, J. J. and Thomas, S. A. (1980) Animal companions and one year survival of patients after discharge from a coronary care unit. *Public Health Reports, 95, 307-312.*

Serpell, J.A. (1991) Beneficial effects of pet ownership on some aspects of human health. *Journal of the Royal Society of Medicine*, 84, 717-720.

Anderson, W., Reid, P. and Jennings, G. l. (1992) Pet ownership and risk factors for cardiovascular disease. Medical Journal of Australia, 157, 298-301.

Robinson: The Waltham Book of Human-Animal Interactions: Benefits and Responsibilities, Pergamon Press, 1995.

Steiger, Brad and Sherry, Animal Miracles-Inspirational and Heroic True Stories, 1999 (call 800 872 5627).

Masson, Jeffrey, Dogs Never Lie About Love, Crown Rivers Publishers, NY, 1997.

Gebelein, Eric, Wilderness as Healer, Thornton Publishing, Littleton, CO, 2001.

The Therapeutic Use of Companion Animals, Clinical Geriatrics, 10:4, April 2002.

American Society for the Prevention of Cruelty to Animals

www.aspca.org

Center to Study Human-Animal Relationships and Environments
www.censhare.umn.edu

The Delta Society
www.deltasociety.org

Eden Alternative
www.edenalt.com

Four Paws Animal Foundation
www.members.aol.com/theeshosh/FOURPAWS.html

Project Pooch Pet Therapy Links
www.pooch.org

Service Dogs
www.dogs.about.com

Barker, Dr. Sandra, *Psychiatric Times,* February 1999.

III ARDS FROM DIFFERENT PERSPECTIVES

What follows are three remarkable stories which show that ARDS can happen to anyone – with devastating consequences.

The first story by Meg Tapucol-Provo is a courageous account of a 42-year-old woman whose joy of pregnancy and delivery was followed by a nightmare of complications related to ARDS. The ARDS was caused by an amniotic fluid embolism to her lungs following a Caesarean section. The story is told by Meg and her husband, Tom, who was with her throughout this ordeal while he cared for their two children and his work. Prior to her illness, Meg worked as a freelance cultural diversity trainer, software trainer and on-camera spokesperson. Meg is the founder of the Northwest ARDS Support Network, an organization that provides outreach and support to ARDS patients and their families. This is an inspiring story with a happy continuation…

MY MIRACLE STORY
by Meg Tapucol-Provo

MEG: The morning of December 28, 1998 was filled with anticipation. I had spent the previous five weeks on complete bed rest in the hospital, and now the day had arrived for our daughter, Karina, to be born. I'd spent both Thanksgiving and Christmas on the high-risk pregnancy floor at Swedish Medical Center in Seattle and was really looking forward to resuming a normal life with my husband, Tom, my two-year-old son, Giancarlo and our new baby.

I looked around at the bare walls and empty windowsill. Just the day before, Tom had taken down the Christmas tree, the lights, the wreath and the stockings. He had packed up the poinsettias that had covered my windowsill. The nurses had joked with us that if there had been a contest for "most festive room," we would have won hands down. At about 9:00 in the morning, my obstetrician performed an amniocentesis on me to check whether Karina's lungs were mature. Thanks to the steroid injections given to me at the beginning of my hospital stay, her lungs had fully matured, although it was still five weeks before her due date. We prepared for the C-section to be performed later in the day. After hours of waiting, we were finally sent to the operating room where I was prepped and draped. The only anxiety I had was about the spinal block. I squeezed my eyes shut and tried to think distracting thoughts—I was only partially successful in blocking out the pain of the big needle going into my lower back. But once I was numb, we were ready to get the show on the road.

A scheduled C-section doesn't have all the drama of a "natural childbirth," but for medical reasons, it's the only birth experience I've had and I've never felt like I missed out. In fact, I appreciated the fact that I was calm and pain-free through both of my deliveries. After Karina was delivered, Tom brought her up to my head and my eyes took in her beauty for the first time. I at once felt love and admiration for this little baby, and relief that our ordeal was finally over.

After I was stitched up, I was wheeled to the recovery room. I had been in there for about 45 minutes when suddenly, I started gasping for breath. "Tom, I can't breathe!"

"Calm down, just try to take deep breaths..." "I can't...I

130

can't...Help me!" One of the doctors came in and started massaging my abdomen, causing me to wince in pain. Then I was out.

I remember waking up again, and this time there appeared to be more people in the room. The person who was massaging my abdomen was really hurting me, and I recall trying to hit him and push his hands away. I also vaguely remember someone trying to put a needle in my neck. I was terrified. Then I was out again. Or at least I have no recollection of what happened next.

Tom: *"Something's wrong!" I yelled to the nurse and the anesthesiologist. One of them took her blood pressure and discovered it was dropping quickly. It was my worst nightmare--she had gone into cardiac arrest. A code was called. Doctors, nurses, respiratory therapists, pharmacists and other support people rushed to the small room on the Labor and Delivery floor. Fortunately, the anesthesiologist had intubated Meg right away so that oxygen could continue getting to her brain. Another doctor was massaging her abdomen to try to get her uterus to clamp down and stop bleeding. It wasn't working--blood was pouring out of her. As soon as her heart stopped they began doing CPR, first with chest compressions, then a defibrillator. For 45 minutes, I watched from where I sat on the gurney just outside the door. With every chest compression and every electric shock, I could see her feet flopping up and down as the doctors desperately tried to save her life. There were multiple IV's in place, unit after unit of blood was being transfused into her, and at one point, someone came running down the hall with blood from Spokane--Meg had wiped out the Puget Sound Blood Center. To say I was in shock would be an understatement.*

I literally saw my life changing at that moment. Things were looking grim--she had undergone resuscitation for 45 minutes with no success. The elation I had felt after the birth of our daughter just an hour earlier was replaced by unspeakable fear and dread. I thought about what my life would be like without Meg. I thought about being a single father with a two-year-old and a newborn. I thought about selling the house, or maybe getting a roommate to help with the payments. I immediately called my brother, Christopher, and my dad, Fred. They rushed to the hospital to be with me.

After about 45 minutes of CPR, someone came up to me and

*gently asked, "Would you like some spiritual support?"
"Absolutely." Things were not looking good. I wondered how long the
doctors would keep trying before giving up." Does it matter what
religion?" "No, just get me anyone." A few moments later, Christine,
one of the chaplains, appeared in the hallway. She began praying with
me--it was the most beautiful prayer I had ever heard in my life. I
remember feeling that she somehow had a "direct line" to God.*

*Two minutes later, from inside the room, I heard the words,
"We've got a heartbeat!" Our prayers had been answered—I couldn't
help but think that we had just witnessed a miracle. When Dad and
Christopher arrived, all four of us went down to the chapel and
continued to pray to God that Meg's life would be spared. We weren't
out of the woods yet. Meg was stabilized, and then brought down to the
Intensive Care Unit. At this point, no one knew what had caused the
cardiac arrest. All they knew was that she was bleeding uncontrollably
and was having coagulation problems (Disseminated Intravascular
Coagulopathy, also known as DIC). They had to pack her nostrils with
gauze because blood was streaming out of her nose and they feared she
would bleed to death. A risky decision was made to bring her to
Interventional Radiology to embolize the bleeding suspects. That
decision was another lifesaving one, because at that point, she would
have probably died within the hour.*

*Over the next several days, she required massive fluid
resuscitation requiring approximately 50 liters of fluid. This resulted in
the swelling of her entire body. She had about 100 extra pounds of fluid
in her and was unrecognizable. Her face had swollen so much that her
features looked like they were flat against her face. Her neck, mouth
and nose were one big blob and her eyes were swollen shut. Her sides
had ripped open because her skin had been stretched beyond the
breaking point.*

*On December 31st, three days after the cardiac arrest,
exploratory surgery was performed. Several liters of clot were
removed, but no active sites of bleeding could be found. A decision was
made to terminate the operation. The doctors told me she had 24
hours. The chaplain was called and the Sacrament of Healing was
administered (formerly known as Last Rites). Miraculously, she made
it through the night, and continued to fight the battle of her life.*

In addition to her bleeding problems, she suffered kidney

failure, liver failure and ARDS (acute respiratory distress syndrome). She was on kidney dialysis for four hours every day to get the extra fluids and toxins out of her system. Her liver was in total distress trying to deal with all the toxins, medications and leftover blood products. She was still intubated and on a ventilator. Things were not looking good.

Meg: The first time I became aware that I was in Intensive Care was six days after I had given birth, on January 3rd. I was trying to open my eyes and I couldn't. *Oh no, I must have left my contacts in my eyes when I had the C-section and now they're stuck to my eyeballs. Great. Now what am I going to do?*

Suddenly, I heard Tom's voice. "Meg, Meg can you hear me?" I nodded my head. "Meg, you're okay. You're in the ICU on a ventilator and it is January 3rd. Don't worry, I'll be right here with you. Now try and get some rest." I slowly became aware of something in my mouth and a tight strap starting at the corners of my mouth and going around the back of my neck. I was mortified.

Being on a ventilator was the single most traumatic thing I experienced during my whole ordeal. I couldn't talk because I had a bite block in my mouth, which was held on by the neck strap. The strap was so tight that it caused indentations in my jaw line. The bite block held the endotracheal tube--a tube that went down my airway and into my lungs. Several times a day, fluid would accumulate in my lungs, causing my breathing to be labored. The only solution was to be suctioned. Anyone who has been on a ventilator knows that suctioning is one of the most dreaded procedures one can experience. A small suctioning tube is placed in the endotracheal tube and pushed down into the lungs. Saline is then put into the suctioning tube and when you feel it in your lungs, you're supposed to start trying to cough. This allows the fluid to be suctioned out of the lungs and you can breathe better. I always dreaded suctioning, but I also felt better after it was done. So I got used to it, but I never liked it.

What I remember from my early days in the ICU was being woken up on a daily basis very early in the morning to be weighed and have a chest x-ray done. I'd go through four hours of dialysis every day and try to sleep through it. Sometimes Tom would come to the hospital first thing in the morning, other days he would be there at lunchtime.

As soon as he'd leave, I'd become enveloped in an anxiety that was almost suffocating. I'd immediately call for a nurse to come to my room just so I wouldn't be alone. They'd try to get me to relax and go to sleep, but it was so difficult. And when I did sleep, there were the dreams.

One very vivid dream I had was that a beautiful dark-haired woman came to my room and said the most wonderful prayer. It was as if an angel had come to me, and I literally heard harps playing in the background. She asked me if I wanted to go to the chapel with her. She made me feel so warm and comforted. In my dreamlike state, I floated through the hallways of Swedish Medical Center until I got to the chapel, but then I couldn't find her. The hallways were dark. In fact, they were more like tunnels. But I wasn't scared, and I felt like everything was going to be okay. I just waited and waited at the chapel doors, and then somehow I ended up back in my hospital bed. Later, I told Tom of my dream and I described the woman I saw. He told me that I was describing Christine, the chaplain who had said the prayer the night of the cardiac arrest. This is one of many dreams that I had while unconscious, but after doing some reading, I believe this dream may have represented a near-death experience.

Through this entire ordeal, my husband was by my side every step of the way. I was terrified and depressed but he did everything he could to keep my spirits up. Had he not been there for me, I don't think I would have made it.

Tom: Fortunately, I had a very understanding employer who made it clear to me that Meg was to take priority over my work. I went to the hospital everyday and became very much a presence in the ICU. Since Meg was unable to communicate, I felt I needed to be her advocate. I wanted to make sure that the doctors and nurses saw her as a person, not just another poor soul on a ventilator. I brought pictures of our family into the room so that the staff could see how she really looked. Meg had also done quite a bit of work as an on-camera spokesperson, so I found a video in which she was confidently explaining bone marrow transplant procedures to potential transplant recipients. I wanted the doctors and nurses to hear her voice. I wanted them to become emotionally connected to her. They did connect with her, so much so that one of the nurses actually had to request not to work with

Meg anymore. Meg was suffering so many setbacks that they began to take an emotional toll on this particular nurse, who had come to care for Meg very deeply.

I was given permission by the nursing supervisor to look at Meg's daily lab results on the computer. I became very familiar with what "normal" levels were for different chemicals in the body and would have daily discussions with the doctors and nurses about Meg's progress. A couple of times, I arrived at the hospital to find that the doctors were about to start a procedure that I knew nothing about. I would insist that they hold off until I was given a thorough explanation of the procedure and understood the risks as well as the benefits.

I wanted to support Meg in every way I could because she was really struggling with keeping her spirits up. I went to the hospital every day, often twice a day. When I was at the office, I would fax her little notes of encouragement. I urged her to look at every small achievement as a victory, and to continue to look forward rather than dwelling upon what had happened. Her mom had given me a prayer for healing, which I brought to the hospital and said with her twice a day. I also said the rosary every day during my half-hour commute to and from Seattle. An acting buddy of hers from the Bay Area had given her a little chrome "meg" that he'd taken off an old Oldsmobile Omega. I put it on my dashboard in front of the speedometer so that all my energy was constantly focused on her and her healing.

Thanks to the Internet, I was able to keep friends and relatives updated on Meg's condition via e-mail. There were about 85 people who received these e-mails, and they in turn forwarded the e-mails to hundreds of others. Meg's name appeared on practically every prayer list in the Seattle area. Hundreds of people were praying for Meg in places as far away as the Philippines, Iceland, Indonesia and Singapore. Old college friends and theatre buddies of Meg's heard about her situation and e-mailed their support. One was a vascular surgeon on Maui who actually ended up giving me a lot of guidance on some of Meg's medical issues. Many of Meg's friends worked in the medical field, either as doctors, nurses or pharmacists. These friends, who I referred to as "Meg's Medical Team," consulted with their own colleagues about Meg's condition. Everyone seemed to agree that it was miraculous that Meg was still alive.

The entire first month was a roller coaster ride. Her

pulmonologist tried taking her off of the ventilator on Day 12, but had to put her back on. We were also waiting for her kidneys to begin producing urine. She needed to be at an output of 1000 cc's before dialysis wouldn't be needed. Unfortunately, her best day was 300 cc's and a couple of days it was less than 50 cc's. I told everyone on the e-mail list to pray for her kidneys to start working. Or, as my brother Christopher put it, "PEE MEG!"

She showed signs of improvement up until Day 14, and her blood came close enough to normal that her hematologist said he'd be signing off. Then on Day 15, she began oozing blood from her C-section incision. Her abdomen became more and more swollen--and the surgeons performed emergency surgery to try and find the problem. Three liters of fluid and old liquefied blood were evacuated from her abdominal cavity. Again there was no evidence of a bleeding site, so her condition could not be corrected. They again had to give her lots of blood and blood factors and other fluids just to keep her pressure up. Her body was in a septic condition. After the surgery, we watched her sink lower and lower. Her surgeon grimly informed us that she again only had 24 hours to live. We stood by as the chaplain again performed the Sacrament of Healing.

Miraculously, with the help of God, the angels watching over her and all the other positive energy she received, she woke up overnight with her blood pressure close to normal! It was fun watching the doctors try to figure out what had happened overnight! When her surgeon came to visit her, his jaw dropped. He knew that there was no medical explanation for Meg's survival

In the middle of the first month, Meg's friend and colleague, Diane Landsinger of Boeing decided she wanted to do something to help. Whenever people asked me what they could do to help, I would answer, "Give blood." Meg had been working with Diane as a contract diversity trainer just prior to entering the hospital, and had also done prejudice reduction training with her for the Anti-Defamation League A World of Difference Institute. Diane wrote an article for the Boeing Lifeline, the company's online health newsletter, explaining Meg's situation, the fact that Meg had already gone through 70 units of blood in just a few days and how the Puget Sound Blood Center was in desperate need of blood. She coordinated a blood drive and 127 Boeing employees who did not know Meg donated blood in her name. Those blood donations combined with blood donations from friends, my co-workers and Meg's co-workers totaled almost 200 units! Diane delivered three posters full of signatures to me and I posted them in Meg's hospital room where she could see them everyday and realize how much people cared.

Meg: Everyday, when I felt depressed and hopeless, I would look at those posters. I was so moved at the caring and generosity of all the donors, and felt that the least I could do was fight the good fight. Those donors gave the gift of life--what better gift could one ask for?

Tom: A couple more setbacks at the end of the first month made me realize that we had a long road ahead of us. In addition to suffering another bleeding episode, Meg ruptured an artery in her abdomen while trying to sit up for the first time, resulting in a massive hematoma in her abdominal wall. The hematoma pushed up into her diaphragm and her lungs and caused further breathing problems. The doctors had never seen a hematoma that huge, which explained their reluctance to give us a prognosis on it. They decided to monitor it with the hopes that it would reabsorb on its own.

Meg and I had made the decision not to let Giancarlo come into the room while she was intubated. We thought it would frighten him too much. I did, however, bring Karina in to see Meg several times. I would hold her close to her mommy and Meg would smile and cry. It was difficult for Meg to go so long without seeing Giancarlo, but we thought it was the best decision at the time. We did not want to further traumatize Giancarlo, who was already having problems dealing with no mommy, a new sister, and full-time day care.

Because it was determined that Meg would probably be on the ventilator for many more weeks, it was decided that she would undergo a tracheotomy, during which an incision would be made in her neck and a breathing tube placed into her trachea. She had been intubated for four weeks. Her bleeding had finally stabilized enough; at this point the trach would be more comfortable for her. Of course, her doctor was required to inform me of the risks involved. He did not paint a very pretty picture, and as a result I was extremely agitated during the surgery, which took longer than they had said it would take. I breathed a sigh of relief when I was informed, three hours later, that the surgery was a success.

Meg: Once the trach was in place, we allowed Giancarlo to come and visit me. It had been four weeks since I'd seen him and I missed him so much. I hoped that he would realize that inside this person with tubes coming out from everywhere, who couldn't talk, who could barely move, and was yellow from jaundice, was the mommy who loved him more than anything. I think he did know that, but I also know that whenever he hears us talking about the hospital, he becomes very quiet and he puts his hands over his ears. He does not want to relive that horror and hates being reminded of it. Being able to see my children was one of the things that kept me going. If not for them and Tom, I might have given up.

Tom: The more aware Meg became, the more difficult it was for her to deal with her condition. She was unable to sleep without drugs, so every night she would ask the nurse for sleep medication. She never really slept more than three hours at a time, and even then, her sleep was not deep and restful. I was afraid she would become addicted to the drugs so I insisted that she avoid certain ones. I even tried to get her to sleep by massaging her feet, which worked! I encouraged others to massage her feet. If the nurses weren't too busy, they did it too.

Meg developed what is known as "ICU Psychosis" in which a patient starts becoming paranoid and anxious. It has to do with a disrupted sleep pattern. The average length of stay in the ICU is one to two days--Meg was there for more than two months. There is activity taking place in the ICU 24 hours a day--nurses coming in and out of the room and alarms going off all the time. On top of all that, Meg had tons of medication in her system. According to one of her night nurses, she went a full month-and-a-half without a good night's sleep.

Meg: As time wore on, I began to wonder if I'd ever get out of the ICU. I dreaded being alone. I hated dialysis. My hands were shaking because of all the drugs in my system, which meant I could no longer write legibly. In order to communicate, I had to point to letters on a piece of paper and spell out what I was trying to say. Sometimes people would try to read my lips, but that was really frustrating, for them and for me.

Sometimes I thought about Jack Kevorkian. It wasn't exactly that I had a death wish, but I occasionally thought that it would be easier to just close my eyes and never wake up. I had been in the ICU for so long. I really didn't see any end in sight. Other times I thought about Christopher Reeve, especially when I had "pop offs" which is when your trach tube becomes disconnected and you can't breathe. I remembered the image of sheer terror that came to my mind when he described that experience in his autobiography, *Still Me*. The first time it happened to me was in the middle of the night. It made me realize just how little control I had over one of the most basic functions of my body--breathing. I frantically tried feeling where the tube should have been connected but I had no idea what I was doing. I panicked. *Oh my God, I'm going to suffocate to death because no one will know that my trach came apart.* But of course they knew. An alarm sounds at the nurse's station when something goes wrong with the ventilator. Within seconds (although at the time it seemed like forever) a respiratory therapist came strolling in and quickly reconnected the tube. The "pop offs" were something I never got used to. Plus, I thought, what if no one was at the nurse's station when the alarm went off? It was too horrifying to think about.

Tom: In early February, the doctors finally determined what caused the cardiac arrest and subsequent DIC, sepsis, and ARDS. Meg had suffered an amniotic fluid embolism (AFE). This is an extremely rare condition in which amniotic fluid somehow gets into the bloodstream and travels to the lungs. The incidence of AFE is 1 in 80,000 and the mortality rate is thought to be as high as 86%. (In fact, because so few women survive AFE, the diagnosis of this condition is usually made during autopsy.) Of the few who do survive, particularly an embolism of the magnitude that Meg survived, relatively few are neurologically intact. Some live in a vegetative state for the rest of their lives. Because Meg had survived not only the AFE, but ARDS, DIC, and sepsis, each of which has relatively high mortality rates, she was known as "The Miracle Patient" at Swedish. She had beaten the incredible odds that were stacked against her. Still, we weren't sure what her quality of life would be once she was able to breathe off the ventilator.

The kidney specialist was beginning to think that maybe Meg's kidneys would never function again. He brought up the possibility of permanent dialysis. He even mentioned the possibility of a kidney transplant down the road. The dialysis access in Meg's neck, which was a central line directly to her heart, was not intended for long-term use and her doctor feared it would become infected. He suggested putting a Gore-Tex shunt in her left forearm to connect an artery to a vein and provide dialysis access. I put him off for about two weeks, because I really believed her kidneys would come back. But finally I had to relent, and surgery #7 was performed to insert the shunt into her arm. Her arm was extremely painful and swollen and she had to sleep with her arm raised for several weeks. I told everyone on the e-mail list to pray for her kidneys. I also obtained a reflexology diagram that showed the part of the feet that affected the kidneys. I massaged that part of her feet every day. The doctors thought I was wasting my time. But by the time the shunt was ready to be used, her kidneys had almost completely recovered, and the shunt was only used twice!

On Sunday, February 21st, we held a prayer vigil for Meg. At this point, she had been in the ICU for 55 days. Even though she was progressing well, we wanted to send a big powerful wallop of prayers and energy to help her turn the corner. There were about 25 people who showed up at our church in Seattle and at least 100 more throughout the United States. My sister, Meegan, and her women's group gathered in Indonesia while her boyfriend, Dave, and his friends joined the prayer vigil from a Buddhist temple in Singapore.

Meg's friend Trish, who lives in Walla Walla, also gathered friends at her house that night to meditate for Meg's greatest good. Trish's friend, Teresa, is a clairvoyant who had been sending Reiki treatments to Meg telepathically. (Reiki is a Japanese form of healing energy.) That night as they meditated, Teresa broke out in a sweat and was weak after the session. She said that so much healing was being pulled that she wondered at the power of their meditation. Trish reminded her that there were many people gathered in prayer for Meg and that explained what she was sensing.

Meg: I remember the night of the vigil very vividly. The nurse who had been assigned to me that night had brought in a couple of movies for me to watch. He knew I had problems sleeping and the movies were something to help pass the time. As usual, I called him to my room over and over again, just to ask him to massage my feet, or hold my hand, or just be there in the room with me so I wouldn't be alone. At one point while I was watching one of the movies, I looked over at the clock and realized the prayer vigil was taking place. I closed my eyes and tried to quiet my thoughts. Gradually, I felt warmth enveloping my body. I knew everything was going to be okay.

Tom: Meg was finally weaned off the ventilator in late February. She was transferred to the renal floor in early March after more than two months in the ICU. As she was leaving in her hospital bed, the entire ICU staff lined the hallways to wish her well. There were so many tears shed, and the amount of love and caring that we felt from the staff was overwhelming. It was a moment we'll never forget.

Meg: I spent two weeks on the renal floor continuing dialysis every other day. It was during this time that I realized my muscles had atrophied. One night I had a dream that I needed to go to the bathroom. Somehow I had pulled myself to the edge of the bed and tried to stand up, and I immediately collapsed to the floor. I laid there in pain for what seemed like an eternity. I couldn't call the nurse because I couldn't get back up on the bed to reach the call button. Thankfully, a nurse finally walked in to check up on me and was shocked to see me lying on the floor.

I was transferred to the rehab floor in mid-March (two-and-a-half months after giving birth) and spent the next month-and-a-half relearning how to walk and take care of myself. It was a grueling schedule, beginning with speech therapy before breakfast, an hour of occupational therapy (OT) and an hour of physical therapy (PT) in the pool before lunch, another hour of OT after lunch and one more hour of PT in the gym in the late afternoon. Once a week the recreational therapist, Lisa, would take a group of us out in the community with our wheelchairs and walkers so that we could get used to the outside world again. We'd go to the Frye Museum, Starbucks, or Baskin-Robbins. Lisa also took a liking to me and offered to use her new Watsu skills on me. Watsu is water massage--Lisa would hold me in her arms in the pool and move me gracefully back and forth through the water. It was an incredibly relaxing feeling, and the PT aides would even turn down the lights and put jazz music on. Everyone there made me feel so special.

I never thought the day would come, but finally, on April 30, 1999, five months and one week after entering the hospital, I was released. The staff gave me a beautiful going away party, decorating the dining room in the rehab unit as well as the door to my hospital room. The table in the dining room was covered with a wonderful spread of food surrounding a delicious looking cake. Lisa had invited everyone who had ever worked with me. All morning, people from all over the hospital came by the party to wish us well. After all that time in the hospital, I had made many friends and had even come to know quite a bit about their personal lives. I was going to miss them, but I was also looking forward to going home and being with my family again.

I continued outpatient physical therapy for eight months at Swedish, then continued my PT program at a nearby health club for another seven months. I slowly graduated from a walker to a cane, and then to walking without a cane. However, I still experienced excruciating pain in my legs from nerve damage that was caused by my illness. As a result, I was unable to be on my feet for more than 10 or 15 minutes at a time. I also had a problem with keeping my food down which lasted for months. I finally went through biofeedback to help me with that and very gradually I regained the ability to keep my food down.

Eight months after I was released from the hospital, I attempted to return to training a couple days a month; however, it was physically very difficult for me without an assistant. Not only would I be exhausted, but also by the afternoon my legs would be screaming with pain because of the nerve damage. Plus, I hadn't bonded with Karina for her entire first year of life. Giancarlo had also been impacted adversely by the tremendous upheaval that had taken place in his life and it was showing in his behavior. I decided to stay at home with them, at least until both were in school. I felt that my life had been spared so that my children wouldn't have to go through life without their mother, and I wanted to maximize the time spent with them.

There are just a couple of residual problems from my ordeal. My abdominal hematoma appears to have stopped reabsorbing and I still look pregnant. And the nerve damage in my legs is permanent. I take medication for the pain in my legs and have been working out at a health club to try to get back into shape. I may not be able to do many of the active things I used to do, such as skiing and playing tennis, but I am learning new ways of being active.

On April 13, 2000, almost a year after I had left the hospital, Tom and I hosted a thank you luncheon at Swedish Hospital for all the folks who had worked with me. We were so grateful to everyone for saving my life and we wanted to show our appreciation. About 65 people showed up and it was so gratifying to be able to see everyone again now that I was healthy. It made everyone feel proud of the work they do. Tom and I also had a very emotional moment when Christine Dickerson, the chaplain who had prayed for me when I had no heartbeat, walked in. We cried tears of joy with this woman who was so instrumental in communicating with God so that my life would be spared. Even though she is a real-life person, she will always be an angel for us.

Needless to say, this was an incredibly life-changing experience for us. When you come so close to death, your priorities change really quickly. When you are fighting for your life, little things that used to stress you out suddenly become unimportant. I am grateful for every day that I'm alive. I'm also grateful that I came out of that harrowing experience relatively unscathed.

Tom: Our faith has never been stronger. This was a gift--God wanted Meg to be here for our family. I cannot even count how many miracles were at work here. If you could have seen all the specialists walking out of Meg's room in the ICU with very baffled looks on their faces! They supported Meg, and God and Meg did the work.

Epilogue: Memorial Day, 2001

It has been two-and-a-half years since my illness. Life has pretty much returned to normal. Giancarlo and Karina both attend Montessori schools in the morning and I spend my days taking care of them and occasionally doing some on-camera and voice over work, designing websites and writing.

I am flipping through my copy of *Simple Abundance* by Sarah Ban Breathnach. This wonderful book contains lessons for every day of the year—lessons that enable one to "encounter everyday epiphanies, find the Sacred in the ordinary, the Mystical in the mundane, and fully enter into the sacrament of the present moment."

On a whim, I turn to the lesson for November 24th, which happens to be the date in 1998 that I first entered the hospital. The lesson is entitled "The Blessing of Health." In it, Breathnach says:

"Health is a priceless gift from spirit that most of us take for granted until we become sick. 'One of the most sublime experiences we can ever have is to wake up feeling healthy after we have been sick,' Rabbi Harold Kushner reminds us in *Who Needs God.* 'Even if it is only relief from a headache or toothache, the health we take for granted most of the time is suddenly seen to be an incredible blessing.' Today, realize if you have nothing else but your health, you are a wealthy woman. If you have a healthy mind, a healthy heart, and reserves of stamina and creative energy to draw on, the world is literally lying at your feet. With your health you have *everything.*"

I turn the page to the lesson for November 25th, and there, at the top of the page, in big, bold letters, are the words, "When You're Sick." Is this pure coincidence? As I read the lesson, a passage I come across summarizes perfectly what I have been feeling:

"If I'd never sustained a head injury ten years ago, I don't think I would have started my own business, written a syndicated newspaper column, or eventually published three books. My nearly two years' arbitrary sabbatical provided me with the opportunity to strike out on a new path after I recovered. Every illness, from a cold to cancer, has a life-affirming lesson for us if we're willing to be taught. It can be simple or profound. Learning to take better care of ourselves in the future in order to stay healthy. Bringing more harmony into our daily affairs. Balancing our need for rest and recreation with the demands of responsibility. Appreciating the subtle nuances of the dark days as well as the light-filled ones. Seeking Wholeness as well as healing. Searching not just for a possible cure, but for the probable cause."

There are still many times that I let little things get to me. I sweat the small stuff more often than I'd like. But there isn't a day that goes by that I don't think about how blessed I am to be here. And I think that I'm still in the process of learning how to relax more. When I'm feeling stressed or blue, I consciously try to bring myself back to the time that I couldn't move, and I was on life support. It gives me a much-needed perspective on life, and reminds me that it's *all* small stuff.

Addendum – Two Years Later

This addendum to Meg's Miracle story, written by Meg, continues the story of her Miracles and the power of Love and Prayer in her life. And I thank her for the impetus she has provided for me to finish this book to bring messages of hope to those persons with ARDS or other critical illness. Also, the families and friends of seriously ill patients will find hope and inspiration herein.
Steve Yarnall, M.D.

A couple of years after my illness, I started doing some research to see if I could learn anything more about ARDS. This is when I found the ARDS Support Center. Through the ARDS Support Center's Pen Pal Circle I met several people who would ultimately lead me on the path I was meant to take.

One person I "met" through the Pen Pal Circle was Dr. Steve Yarnall. He mentioned that he was writing a book and wanted stories from ARDS survivors. He only wanted about 500 words, and I had written about 2500 words, but I figured I'd give it a shot. Imagine my surprise when I found out that not only was he inspired by my story, but he lived only 30 minutes away from me! We made plans to meet for dinner at Salty's at Redondo, a wonderful seafood restaurant on the Puget Sound, a mile away from my home. Steve, his wife Lynn and their daughter Kim laughed and cried with Tom and me that night at dinner. We shared all those common experiences that only ARDS survivors and caregivers can truly understand. He was the first ARDS survivor I met in person. Steve, Lynn, Tom and I have since become dear friends.

Another friend I made online was Carrie Walker-Bookless. I also read her story on the Pen Pal Circle and noticed that she had been a patient at Harborview Medical Center. I was looking for local people to reach out to, and had she not mentioned the name of the hospital she was at, I would probably not have written to her. Initially, she seemed somewhat reluctant to talk about something that had caused so much pain in her life, but little by little, after exchanging several e-mails, she began to open up. Steve, Lynn, Tom and I met Carrie, her husband, Tod, and her son Alex at their condo in Bellevue for dinner. Again, it was such a wonderful experience for all of us to meet others who had been through the traumatic experience of battling ARDS and surviving it.

Several get-togethers followed—a play date with Carrie, Alex, my daughter Karina, and me. A barbecue at our home. And I began to realize that this was something that was benefiting all of us. All of us were finally able to connect with others who had been through something that no one else could truly understand. Being in a coma. Being on a vent. The hallucinations. Being the caregiver and enduring weeks of not knowing what was going to happen. Finally someone else understood!

After months of talking with another online friend, I took the plunge. Eileen Rubin Zacharias, the founder and president of the ARDS Foundation of Illinois had contacted me because she read my story on the Pen Pal Circle and was trying to connect me with another woman who had developed ARDS after childbirth. Eileen and I started emailing back and forth, and after sharing all of our common ARDS survivor experiences, found that we had much in common beyond that, including two small children ages 5 and 3. When I told her I was thinking of starting an outreach and support group in the Northwest, she provided me with a wealth of information. I didn't want to duplicate her efforts; rather, I wanted to focus on regional in-person support and have my website provide links to the vast Internet resources already available.

The Northwest ARDS Support Network website went online in November 2001. We are currently operating under the fiscal sponsorship of the American Lung Association of Washington. We've had our first official ARDS Survivors Potluck, which was an amazing gathering of survivors and caregivers. We all shared our stories and looked forward to getting together again. In fact, just a month later, we did get together again, at the American Lung Association Breathe Easy Breakfast. We plan on having regular get-togethers, and on supporting each other in any way we can.

We also, unfortunately, were the bearers of devastating news when Carrie, one of the people who inspired me to start the Northwest ARDS Support Network, passed away unexpectedly at the age of 31 on December 30, 2001. Little did Steve, Lynn, Tom and I know that when we attended her holiday/housewarming on December 15th, that we'd be attending her memorial celebration in the same home less than a month later. Although Carrie wanted the memorial to be a celebration of her life, we were saddened that someone we came to know through the shared experience of ARDS had had her life taken away from her at such a young age, leaving behind a husband and a young son.

As far as my health goes, I still have the nerve damage in my legs, which probably will never go away. And my asthma did worsen after the ARDS, but it's not too bad. The one thing that really bothered me was the rectus sheath hematoma that made me look six months pregnant. It never completely reabsorbed on its own, and I was resigned to looking pregnant for the rest of my life.

Then in 2001 I noticed a lump just to the left of my belly button. I talked to my surgeon about it and he said it was an incisional hernia. I had had so many abdominal surgeries during the time I was ill that the fascia had become weakened and developed a hole where the incisions intersected. It just so happened that the hernia could not be repaired without also removing the hematoma! I was ecstatic! The doctors would never have operated on me just to remove the hematoma on its own because it was not life-threatening and the surgery would have been too risky. But the hernia HAD to be repaired, and there was no other way to do it without removing the hematoma! Boy did I luck out!

So on April 9, 2002, I went back to Swedish Medical Center to have the hernia repaired and the hematoma removed. We requested the anesthesiologist who saved my life—what an emotional reunion that was! The surgeon who would be performing the procedure had also been involved in my care three years ago. Almost everyone involved in this surgery was intimately aware of all the details of my case three years before—this was very important to us. It's funny--I had no fear at all about this surgery. I was just thinking about the outcome—that I'd finally look somewhat normal again, and not have this constant reminder of my illness every time I'd look down and see my distended abdomen.

Tom, on the other hand, was extremely nervous, and understandably so. Almost every surgery I had during the two months I was in the ICU was an emergency surgery, and he never knew whether I'd come out alive. So even though intellectually, he knew this was a very low-risk surgery, emotionally it was difficult to get past all of the feelings from before. Fortunately, his brother Christopher distracted him for the three hours I was in surgery. They ate Greek food, drank coffee, looked at Ferraris, BMWs and exotic sports cars. They came back, got a private family room at Swedish, played cards and watched TV. It also eased Tom's mind when a nurse informed Tom an hour into the surgery that everything was going just fine.

Since I am writing this, you have probably figured that the surgery was a success. Yes it was. But beyond that, a very special thing happened in the hospital—something that made me feel like I've come full circle.

Several people who I did not know came to my room. One was a Labor and Delivery nurse who said to me, "You probably don't remember me, but I was in the room when you coded. I had heard you were in the hospital and I just want to say I'm so glad you made it. It's a miracle you're here." Another was a phlebotomist who came to draw my blood. He looked at my name and said, "You probably don't remember me, but I came to your room in the ICU many times to draw your blood, but you were in a coma. There were hundreds of us in the Lab who were praying for you." I actually did vaguely remember this man, because he would prick my finger and test my bleed times (the length of time it takes your blood to clot) and during that time in the ICU, when I was having severe coagulation problems, he'd sit there for about 25 minutes, just waiting and waiting. He told me how happy they all were that I had pulled through.

Another person who came to my room was one of the anesthesiologists on staff at Swedish. He actually came to my room to take out my epidural, which was being used for steady infusion of pain medication. Later that day, he came back and reintroduced himself. He said, "Your name looked familiar, and then I remembered, Dr. Woodland had called me to assist at your code." So we talked for a long time about that night and what it was like. He said to me, "Do you know what the chances are of you having normal kidney function after what you went through? Almost zero. Do you know what the chances are of you having normal brain function after what you went through? Almost zero. You are a miracle!"

It's heartening that even after three-and-a-half years, all these people still remember me. They recall with great clarity all the details of what happened to me. One likes to think they're not "just another patient." How many thousands of patients do these people see over the years? But yet, they remembered me, and even went out of their way to come to my room and wish me well. That, in itself, is a small miracle. And I would like to think that these little miracles will continue to happen for the rest of my life—a life made possible not only by the wonderful staff at Swedish Medical Center, but by prayer, and most of all, love.

****

FROM CRISIS TO CREATION
by Eileen Rubin Zacharias

Next is the story of a female attorney whose crisis of ARDS led to the creation of the ARDS Foundation of USA. Married for only a year, Eileen was a healthy thirty-three year old woman when she noticed subtle symptoms which soon developed into full-blown ARDS with not-so-subtle complications. Here's a message of hope in the face of apparent hopelessness.

My story begins with lower back pain, which progressed for about five days until I went to an internist. She did a complete exam, but ordered no tests and sent me home with muscle relaxants. Five days later, the pain was so bad and in addition, had moved to my chest (obviously the ARDS had settled in). I saw her associate who did another exam but still ordered no tests and sent me home with more pills.

The next morning, at five am, I called, spoke to the associate and told him that I could not breathe. He told me to call back at ten am when my doctor was in. I did that but my doctor said that since I had been seen the day before she would not see me. I was on an HMO. Later that day, I went to another internist. By the time I got there, my blood pressure was 70/50. I could not drive, could barely walk. The doctor did blood and ordered a chest x-ray. He gave me the option of going to the ER. I was hesitant, because of the HMO. I had heard of the "not medically necessary" statement from going to the ER previously with a migraine.

"I think I'm dying..."

The following morning, when my new internist got my blood results back, he called and ordered me to the ER, telling me and my husband that I was very sick, my white count was three times higher than normal. I was admitted directly into MICU and by that evening, my kidneys failed. My lungs, of course, were getting progressively worse and by Sunday morning, I could not breathe. My last words to my mother were, "I can't breathe, I think I'm dying." The internist told my mother that I was just agitated and reluctantly went into to check on me due to her insistence. Of course, I was in respiratory arrest; my family was pushed out of the room and I was intubated. Hours later, the doctors came out and told them about the ARDS.

I have absolutely no memory of the time that I was in a coma, about four weeks. My family and friends were at the hospital everyday, often all day. Friend's of my parents and siblings were there everyday. More distant relatives also came. At 10 days to two weeks in, they had a meeting with my family and told them that if I did survive, I would never get off the vent. They said that they needed to start thinking about not if, but when to take me off the vent as it would be a quality of life issue. My parents brought in some doctors from other hospitals to do a consult. One doctor from Northwestern told my parents that they were writing me off too soon. He gave them hope and he gave them his pager and urged them to call with questions, which they did.

When I came out of my coma, I was taken off morphine almost "cold turkey". At the same time I was transferred to the respiratory floor, which threw me into a hospital psychosis (psychotic episode). For about three days, I lay mostly awake, eyes bulging and my hands shaking involuntarily. When my neurologist reintroduced my morphine, I was basically fine. I was told that I was the easiest spinal tap because I was completely still and at only 82 pounds, did not have much skin to go through.

It gets worse...

My next five weeks, I was alert enough to remember everything. My lungs collapsed a second time, requiring three more chest tubes and I remember them putting them in. I recall everyone's faces, how concerned they were and I was thinking that it did not seem like such a big deal. I felt bad that the respiratory therapist had to bag me the whole time because it seemed like a long time. Likewise, I needed eight blood transfusions and I got a lot of apologies about it because they said how uncomfortable it was. But it did not bother me a bit. On the other hand, only a day after they removed my main line, I developed a secondary pneumonia in my trach, and I went ballistic when they had to poke me for the IV. I have very bad veins. And I think that sometimes the minor things are your breaking point.

While on the respiratory floor, I had an impossible time getting off the vent. I have told people that getting off the vent was the hardest thing that I have ever done in my life--harder than law school, harder than the bar exam, harder than doing a murder jury, more difficult than my divorce from my first husband. I had real panic attacks for the first time in my life. I stopped trying to get off the vent because every day that I put forth some sort of effort, something horrible would happen. I felt like I'd take a step forward and three steps back. I remember that I felt like there was no light at the end of the tunnel. I resented that every day the doctors would come into my room and tell me that I was going to walk out of the hospital. I was certain that I would not.

Anyway, one day, I realized that if I was going to have children, which I had been trying to do prior to getting sick, I was going to have to get off the vent. One of the biggest motivating people was my occupational therapist who, unlike family, could push me, albeit gently, to make progress. I wanted to make her proud. And so, I remember the day, a Sunday, when I decided to make a conscious effort to get off the vent. And that very night, when I was all alone and my inclination was to call for my nurse to tell her, as I usually did, that I was anxious, I instead took those deep breaths and made it through the night. The next day, I was already reducing my settings.

Someone asked me if I ever asked G-d for help in getting off the vent. And although I believe in G-d, it never even occurred to me to ask G-d for help. I was happy that many people of all different beliefs, as my family told me, were praying for me. One man, who knew me from when I was a young child from Synagogue when I was with my family, he was praying for me every day. In fact, he still includes me in his daily prayers.

"The patient from hell"

When I got moved to the respiratory floor, the doctors told my family to bring things in to make me feel more at home. One day, my pulmonologist came in the room, announced that I was watching too much TV and changed the TV station to the hospital music station. I was just out of my coma and was so weak that I could not lift my arms/hands to find the call button/TV changer. For some reason, my family was not there. I remember feeling so desperate, unable to communicate in any manner, and just wanting to have the television on to distract me. Eventually, I just dozed off. When I woke, my parents were in the room and the TV was on. I felt relieved. They did bring in a CD player and bought some music that I would normally enjoy. I listened to one CD twice. For me, it was not relaxing, it was not a comfort. The TV was my great distraction and I had it on all day and all night. And believe me, in the summer, there is no good TV on.

When I was getting a little better, my room became too cluttered. I became the patient from hell. I wanted all of that stuff my husband and family brought for me to comfort me to be taken away. I kept a few things and some pictures of my pets. I recall, too, over the Fourth of July holiday, being so concerned for the dogs because the people in my neighborhood not only shoot fireworks but also shoot off guns (cop neighborhood...my husband is a police officer). Also, I was sick during Chicago's heat wave where over nine hundred people died from the weather. It was very surreal to hear about all of those deaths while I was in the hospital. Our house had no air, and I was overly concerned for the animals, two dogs and two cats.

I sent away all of the flowers. The smell bothered me and there were just too many. I did not want visitors who were not immediate family or very close friends, because up until the last week. I would not look at myself in the mirror so why should I subject others to do so. But I wanted my mother there all day long. I'd give her a break in the evening when others would come. My husband was given one day off by the police department and he looked like the walking dead, doing police work all day and coming to the hospital at night -- same with my brothers and sisters. My father stopped working all together for six weeks and my mother did not go back to work until I had been home for over a month.

Love, Prayer, and Humor

I am convinced that the love and prayers of family and friends were crucial to my survival. I am also convinced that the fact that my family was there at the hospital all of the time made my physicians more accountable for everything that they were doing.

My recovery once out of the hospital was amazingly quick because I was so focused on getting better so that I could start to try to get pregnant. (six months later) I think that having something positive to focus on is key. Not to say that I did not experience depression at a later date as a result of my ARDS experience. (That happened at my two-year anniversary.) I did not work for almost a year and then only part time. I will probably always work part time, not because I can't work full time, but because I want to be here to raise my kids, I am too high stress, and my health is too important.

I don't think we added humor to the equation until my last week when it was clear I would be walking out of the hospital. But now I try to look at some of those horrible memories that I have with humor. I am an identical twin and when people ask how to tell us apart, we say, "I'm the one with the hole in my neck." When I don't remember something, I tell people that if it was BC (Before Coma), I am off the hook. When discussing the kids with other moms, I tell them that I am more sympathetic to the whole diaper thing since I am probably the only one I know who remembers diapers. (I now have two daughters, ages three and five.)

In addition to family, friends, and strangers, the people who were with me at the hospital were just incredible regarding encouraging my recovery. My ICU nurses and my primary nurse on the respiratory floor were outstanding. Many of the other nurses were kind, caring and encouraging. I felt like they were friends. The first time that I was able to walk out of the room past the nurses' station, everyone cheered like I was a one-year old walking for the first time. When I had several panic attacks, it was the nurses who sat with me, calming me down, sometimes for as long as a half hour while I shook.

When I go back to the hospital, most of them still remember me, as I do them, and they even remember the room that I was in. And many of the doctors were kind and compassionate above-and-beyond the call of duty. Often, they would come by as a "social call" to see how I was as they did not need to see me at that particular time. They would delight at my progress. Only a couple of the doctors were annoyed at how high functioning I was because I had too many questions. Some would just turn their backs and walk out. When I was strong enough, I would throw things to try to get their attention. The nurses would always come in later and wonder out loud how the pad of paper or the stuffed animal got on the ground close to the door.

I have no nightmares as a result of this. My pulmonologist, who told me that I almost died at least five times, doubted that I would remember as much as I do. I was on an enormous amount of morphine and fentynal and other related drugs. But my last five weeks are vivid to this day. My neurologist told me that I am the sickest person who he has ever seen who had lived. I have some of my typewritten reports and every so often, read them to remember where I was at and where I am now. I do it as a positive thing and not to dwell on the negative.

When I got home from the hospital, my insurance company rejected each and every medical bill because the doctor that admitted me was not an HMO doctor. (all of the referring specialists were part of the HMO) My bills were around $500,000. It took me over six months of fighting with the insurance company to get them to pay every last cent. I know the insurance companies don't care that in that weakened state, the patient must now deal with all of this. It does make it harder to move on with life and get healthy.

Six Years Later

My life is better now. It has not all been easy, but I have a fuller life than I ever would have had if my life had not been interrupted by ARDS. I completely revaluated everything in my life and pared down many areas.

Life does have a way of working out even when it seems hopeless. This supports Nietzsche's dictum, "what doesn't kill you makes you stronger." Life will have its share of frustrations. Sometimes having the right attitude makes things happen or be easier to bear. Where there is life, there is hope.

ADDENDUM - Humor in Everything

I just thought of something that has amused me in the years that have past since I was ill. For a long time after I got out of the hospital, I was a little obsessed with the thought that the doctors spoke to my family about donation of my organs-since they said that I almost died at least five times, not such a ludicrous thought-but it bothered me. Everyone told me no, but I did not really believe them.

But then it occurred to me why they never would have mentioned that. My organs appeared shot. There were problems with probably every organ except my eyes. They would not even want my organs. And when I realized that, my obsession about that ended. And now, the whole thing makes me laugh. You see, there is humor in everything!

CARRIE'S COURAGE AND HUMOR
by Carrie Walker Bookless

Next is the story of a young mother who developed ARDS with subsequent pulmonary fibrosis (scarring of lungs) and died while waiting for a lung transplant. Carrie relates her conquest of alcoholism and exhibits her remarkable sense of humor in the face of horrendous stresses. You will laugh and cry as you read the account of what was to be the last days of her life, which ended on December 30, 2001.

Prelude to the accident

I was 22 and was the daytime manager of a popular bar and grill. I had been dating someone for 2 years and had just recently broken up with that person. He had been an addict / alcoholic and I myself was a heavy binge drinker. It did not make for a pretty relationship and often resulted in some pretty serious fights. My parents had just flown out to Florida to go to Disney World on their first vacation by themselves in many many many years. It was a Tuesday night and my parents wanted me to stay at their place to keep an eye on their four other kids. I came by after work, and made sure they were all fed, but figured the two in high school wouldn't likely throw a party, so I was going to go out with a cook from my work to celebrate my long awaited break up from Mr. Nasty. My grandmother lived in a guest home behind my parents, so I thought it was pretty safe to go out.

We went to this great little gay dive bar in the Broadway area. They were having a transvestite contest that evening and it all just sounded like a lot of fun. I remember dancing with some very tall women and my friend met up with a young man there. When things calmed down after the show, we 3 decided to head down to the Pioneer Square district of Seattle and attend the last of the Mardi Gras festivities of Fat Tuesday. I recall driving down the hill and parking the car, but that's as much as I recall of the last hour and a half of my healthy life.

The Accident

This is what I was told. We left the bars around 1:30 am when they were clearing everyone out for the night. We started across the street. My friend and another person we were with, were ahead of me. A truck hit me. I got caught in his undercarriage and was drug up the street 50 ft till people forced him to stop. No one recalls whether we were crossing with or against the light, no one, meaning hundreds of people. The truck driver never saw me in the crosswalk. He thought the sound of my body, thumping the ground, was his muffler coming loose.

I arrived at the hospital with multiple fractures in my neck, broken femur, fractured ribs, and a head injury. Probably something I forgot, but I forget a lot of things. My heart and breathing had stopped at the scene and I had been given CPR by my friend. In the ambulance I was given an adrenaline shot to get my heart going again. My body wasn't cooperating. They stabilized me at the hospital finally and everyone thought I would be ok. Not so. I developed ARDS, gained over a hundred pounds in water weight, and had to have my brain drained, due to fluid from a subdural hematoma. I spent about 2 months in an induced coma. I was intubated and on a ventilator for over 8 weeks plus another month and a half on a trach and two more on the rehab floor. I spent just a couple days short of 5 months in the hospital. I went in Feb 23, 1993 I believe and left about on the 21st of July. That may be backwards or mixed up a bit, but first week of the 20's in each month either way.

ARDS

But what about the ARDS you say? Well, it nearly killed me many times. I had over 20 chest tubes placed into my chest. I was one of the worst ARDS patients they had ever had at that time. My pulmonary team tried new things on me, they had only theorized over before, because the likelihood of my living wasn't what they considered a reality. My family was called in time and time again to say goodbye to me. I was given my last rites. If the one thing I have remembered about my life is that what happened to me, helped others to live, this will be enough. I can thank Dr Steinberg and Dr Hudson for that.

My lungs were extremely damaged from scarring. I functioned

on what equaled to less than one lung. But I functioned. I didn't enjoy walking up hills, stairs were a pain, and I could never go scuba diving. I left the hospital on no oxygen, a walker and my life. That was the best gift I ever received till the birth of my son.

ICU Recollections

When I was getting better, my parents put a print on the ceiling for me. I stared endlessly at the ceiling. It was the only thing I could look at. I had braces on my neck and could not turn to look at anything. At one time I had apparently 3 braces on my neck, and another time had a halo drilled in my head, I am told anyway. Ick. Glad I wasn't aware of that at least. Or the tube stuck in the back of my head to my brain. Well the print was a lovely print I was familiar with of a local marina and boats. But my morphined brain kept hallucinating the boats turning into creatures and diving at my face. I knew this wasn't real, but it wasn't very pleasant either. I was happy when it fell off the ceiling onto my head, and they couldn't get it to stick back up. Of course that left the huge bloodstain on the ceiling to view again - another plus of ICU living.

My parents brought in music for them to play to me. My own music but…upbeat and danceable and so annoying during my ordeal, it made me want to climb out of my skin. Where were my Enya tapes?

They put casts on my ankles thinking this was a good thing. I had been in bed for so long, that my ankles were holding my feet in a ballet stance. They thought, "Golly, she's in excruciating pain right now, lets add to it. Let's bend her deforming ankles in an unpleasant angle, cast them up, while her water retention jumps up and make her all betta." My legs swelled over the casts and the ignoramus' waited a couple days, before they relented and took the damn things off. A week or two later, they apparently forgot what happened and tried it again. Had I been able to speak, they would have had an earful. They did get an earful a month and a half later when I could talk.

Yes, they also put me in the CHAIR. What kind of nightmarish beast thought this up? I know, I know. I did need it. But you gain 100+ lbs in water weight, go from 115 lbs to 200 something, then to 70 something in less than 3 weeks and shove your butt onto a hard chair for therapy and tell me how you feel. Not to mention the horror of 3 nurses trying to wriggle your 3 months unwashed body on a thin plastic sheet onto a chair, hooked to a million IV's tubes, catheters and other toys.

Eventually I graduated to a trach. Suction horrors plenty. Hyperventilating constantly in sheer fear. Dying for an ice chip from the Nazi water controllers. After what seemed like years, they moved me out of ICU to not-so-intensive care. I only spent a couple weeks there watching soap operas.

I finally got to the Rehab floor. I had to rebuild nonexistent muscles before I could walk again. But I got better fast. 2 months and I was out. Finally… I think they finally let me out because I could talk again.

Residual Effects-"ARDS Leftovers"

I thought my head problems were brought on by the head injury. After reading other stories, I realize it was probably more the ARDS and it's effects and lack of oxygen on the brain. I have problems with thinking in general, and interactions with people. This, I am happy to say, improves with time. By exercising your brain, it starts working a bit better. I may never overcome, however, my language skill problems. I lose words, can't make my mouth say words, and may say exactly the opposite of what I mean. I say "no", when I thought I said "yes". I say "hamburger", when I mean "horse", and am sure I said horse. This drives my husband up the wall, as you can imagine. I can't recall the word I just said. Or I just simply can't find any words at all to make a simple sentence. This has happened many times just today. I forget what I was talking about the minute I said it. I black out in the middle of a conversation with my husband and have no idea what we were discussing.

For at least three years, I had very few emotions. I felt no love, little happiness, and very rare joy. The only emotion I seemed truly capable of was anger. I had a lot of anger. Things have improved by far, but I still feel like I am just getting the residual effects of emotions.

I am writing this at 3 in the morning. I have sleeping problems. I have nightmares. The second I fall asleep, I start dreaming and wake up often, to only go back to sleep and dream some more. I rarely get any real sleep without medication and I stopped taking medication some years ago. I became aware of my addictive nature to medication at a young age, so declined pain medication a couple weeks after I started physical therapy. I still felt the pain, I just didn't care that I felt it. It didn't seem worth the possibility of getting hooked on expensive drugs.

That knowledge didn't stop my decline into the abyss of alcoholism however. I am now a 4-year sober member of AA. It took till I was 26, with two DUIs and a toxic reaction to a Seabreeze for me to get the picture, that it was definitely time for me to quit drinking. I wasn't a maintenance drinker, but when I did go out drinking, I went out drinking. I was 105 lbs at my heaviest and 5ft tall. I would sit down and drink 10 double 7/7's on a regular basis. It is amazing I would wake up in the morning at all.

More ARDS leftovers: My impulsive behavior. I no longer had a fear of death and did very stupid things. This included a 3-month trip to Europe to get away from my family and their nagging. I decided to go and 2 weeks later was there. The only reason I didn't take off the very second I thought it up, was I had to get a passport first and some luggage. I did make some last minute plans for 2 weeks of the trip but just took some travel books with me and winged the rest of it.

I treated men like disposable lighters for a long time. Most of them were cheap and were only there to light a little fire. Some were the 25-cent brand and only were good for one light. It was all just a game to me. On the outside I seemed well adjusted to all that I went through. I was really a horrible mess suffering Post-traumatic distress. I had very little sleep through the nightmares, regretting my pathetic romantic relationships.

I slowly got better. Little by little. The best thing I ever did was to quit drinking. Through AA I actually got much of the therapy I needed. I was able to apply much of what I learned from others there to my life and make it better. I learned to shut up and to listen to others. I am not perfect and I still do very stupid things. I at least try to stop those behaviors when I spot them.

Grandmother

When they finally moved me to the rehab floor I was talking slightly and was able to sit up and feel slightly more human. I finally took on the task of asking my mother a question that had been on my mind for over a month. "Where is my grandmother?" I asked her if she were dead, being the only reason I knew that would keep her from seeing me. She had passed away while I was in the coma. This was the woman who practically raised me. We had lived next to each other since I was 5 years old. I recall a couple weeks before my accident having to once again go see my grandmother at the local hospital because she had another mild stroke and seizure.

I recall thinking to myself, "Please God, I can't bare seeing her die. Don't make me witness that." I had gotten my wish and I was not happy about it at all. I felt cheated from being able to say goodbye. My mother told me that she assured my grandmother that I was getting better and after she did, she passed away.

The New Challenge

Five years ago I started getting sick again. It was a slow decline. I developed fibrosis of the lungs of unknown origin. It might be caused by the ARDS damage, might not, or may just be amplified by the damage. For the past 4 plus years I have been on oxygen 100% of the time. Spending much of my winters in one hospital or another with pneumonia or some other lung problem.

Up until May of 2001 I was on 6 liters. Unfortunately I became ill again and never recovered. By late June I could no longer care for my son on my own. I couldn't pick him up to change his diapers, get him in or out of his crib or bend over to pick things up that he had dropped. I could no longer do housework or make myself meals. I could barely stand at all for any period of time. Over the summer one of my brothers came and helped me, but when he went back to school in the fall, my mother had to take over. She watches my son and my two nieces at our home. She has her hands full.

I am now on 9 + liters of oxygen to survive. This means very little going out of the home, because I cannot get enough oxygen from portable tanks for any length of time. When I do go out, it is with the aid of a wheelchair, because I cannot walk on so little oxygen. Having to use a public restroom is too much of a nightmare to describe. I usually feel as though I am experiencing a heart attack getting to the pot and from there back to the person who is in charge or pushing me around in the chair.

By the beginning of summer, I knew I could not go on as I was anymore. I decided to try to get on the transplant list finally. My doctors have been recommending it for three years, but I resisted it due to my poor reactions to Steroids, in which you must be on for rejection purposes. On one med I go insane within days of taking it, and all my joints swell up, defeating the anti inflammatory function of it. The other med, that I can use instead, causes severe depression over a period of time, weight gain, acne, and many more lovely effects. For along time I didn't think it was worth it, but I finally got too sick to have any other option. I will die soon without a lung transplant. I may die soon after the transplant from many possible complications, but we know I will die soon without the opportunity.

To get on the list you have to go through all sorts of testing. They want to be sure that if they give you lungs, you are not going to die right away of something else. There is such a shortness of donor lungs, they just can't chance to waste any. It seems heartless, but it wouldn't be a problem if more people were open with their families about their wish to donate their organs. The majority of people waiting for lungs die waiting. Due to the severity of my illness, this is quite a possibility for me. I may have waited too long.

I should have been on the lung transplant list in early September of 2001, but came up against another obstacle. For the first time in my life, my pap smear came back abnormal. The biopsy showed I had buildups of tissue that contained cells that are considered pre-cancerous. I was scheduled for a procedure in late October. During all this time, I could not be on the transplant list. My doctor tells me that the situation is so mild and my condition with the meds I take, being what it is, if we did the procedure, it would only come back, needing another and another. She thought that the likelihood that it would get worse was smaller than the damage that we would create to my body by doing this procedure multiple times. It was decided that we should leave it alone and just keep an eye on it every 4 months. This was great news. This also could have been expressed to the transplant team and me three weeks previous to this on the phone, when they first got the results of the biopsy. I was deeply angry that I had waited an extra three weeks for nothing. Three weeks may not seem like much, but in transplant time, it could mean everything.

In September, I was the only 5' O+ person waiting for lungs in my category. My size limits the amount of donors I have. The donor must be about the same in stature, otherwise the lungs won't fit. So my donor will likely be another very small woman. This rules out the majority of men donors. This can either make my wait quick, or amazingly long. I just met with my pulmonary doctor and I am now not the only small person, but there are 2 more ahead of me in the 5'3" range. She is unsure of the blood type however. I can only hope that they are also not O+ or I could be waiting forever. The average wait is 9 months in the Northwest. This beats the national average of 18 months. Most of the people I know on the list have waited 2 to 3 years. I guarantee I do not have a couple years to sit around left.

Just before I started noticeably getting sick, I quit drinking. This was not all voluntary. I received my second DUI. The first one I received when I was 24 for forgetting to turn my lights back on after pumping gas at a very bright station in the middle of the night. Someone had knocked their beer over on my lap and I smelled to high heaven. The Breathalyzer read very high, but this we deemed was probably from my lung damage more than the possibility that my levels were actually as high as it read. At the time of the first DUI, I could have half a cocktail, wait a half hour, and then breathe into a Breathalyzer and it would read well above legal drinking limits. I know this because we tested it, both on one of those bar entertainment ones and with an actual one, out of curiosity. I had however been drinking and took the DUI and plead guilty. I figured I did the deed and might as well face up. I had to be on probation for 2 years.

One month short of the 2 years, I received my second DUI. This time I got pulled over after drinking, because someone stole my rear license plate. I knew someone had done so, but in my obvious high intellect, thought what the heck, I'll go out with friends and drink. I drank with my usual binge elegance and probably had 7 to 9 double bourbons with and without 7-Up. This time I was trashed, had a blood test instead of taking the breathalyzer, which had I done so, I probably could have fought and got the thing dropped. I however realized that I probably did have a drinking problem and it was time to fess up to all that entailed. I took the deferred, which meant 2 years of treatment center, a few courses, a lot of fines, and 2 mandatory years of AA meetings twice a week.

Soon after the DUI I started really getting sick. I spent over a month in a hospital and from that point on really required oxygen almost all the time. After the first year of treatment and AA meetings, they allowed me to cut down and do most of my treatments one on one or by phone so as not to expose me to illnesses of other patients. TB and illness is rampant in the alcoholic world. They also allowed me to do one meeting a week for the same reasons.

My husband and I found a wonderful group that is both AA and Al-anon. They focus on couples and families. It is the best thing that ever happened to me. I get AA help and we as a couple get free couple therapy from others just like us. It and the couples in it, are probably the number one reason my husband and I are dealing with this whole situation as well as we are. It's not pretty. We still fight, but we can eventually talk it out. We have the resources, sometimes it just takes a while to use them, but we eventually do. I haven't had a drink in over four and a half-years going on five in Feb of 2001 so I guess that says a lot.

It's because of the sanity I found in AA that allowed me the ability to have a higher source. I was pretty bitter many many years for many many reasons. After coming to AA I stopped blaming God for problems. Though this wasn't often much of a problem. My biggest problem was probably the finger I often held in the sky asking what else he thought he had for me. I was a bit cocky after the accident. Maybe that's why I was thrown this loopy loo. Anyway, I started thanking God everyday for giving me another day. It has made me a much nicer person to be around, not to mention a whole lot happier.

Everyday I wake up, I am truly happy for being given another chance to smile at my son and to hold my husband's hand.

8-31-02 Hello all (Eighteen months later)

This is Carrie looking realistically, yet hopefully, at a future of uncertainty as she prepares for a double lung transplant - if it should become available.

S. Yarnall, MD

I just wanted to update everyone on the progress of things. I am now on the transplant list waiting for 2 new lungs. It could come at any time. We are excited as well as scared out of our minds. I'm very tired these days. Tired of living, or rather existing, as I have been. I am excited at the thought I might be given a second chance at a few good years with my husband, child and family and friends. I'm scared to death that I may wake up sicker than now. Which is one possible outcome of transplant surgery. It may take a week or 2 years waiting. More than ever before in my life do I need support and a friendly word of encouragement through this. Your prayers are welcomed. I also know Tod will need an ear now and then. I do not fear death luckily. I got over that years ago with my accident. I do however ache thinking of leaving my husband and son alone. It is a heartbreak I cannot explain or want anyone else to have to understand ever.

I just want everyone to know now how much I care and love you all and not to forget that. Here is hoping the next time I send out an email including so many it will be sent from a veranda eating breakfast in Nice, France with Tod and Alex telling you of our adventures.

...Carrie's concern for others in spite of her own problems...

I would love to make you a quilt for your upcoming addition to the family. I'm afraid I cannot promise it by November however. I still do not have my sewing machine up in action and all my fabrics are packed away downstairs. I have a donation quilt due by the 15th of November to attend to first. It's for a project donating blankies to children of fallen fire fighters and police in New York. Let me know if this is still ok and if you had any druthers on style of the quilt you would like.

Take Care and I will be in touch soon,

...and finally, a simple message of sorrow....

12-31-01 This is Carrie's husband, Tod. Carrie passed away last night.

ADDENDUM - Views on God and Religion

Here is a copy, minimally edited, of Carrie's views on God as she wrote them in the last month of her life. I've left intact Carrie's graphic way of criticizing those who think God is part of an organized religious structure. She calls us to give thanks to God for each day of life and to help others as a priority over sitting in a church singing hymns (although she says this far more bluntly).

God?

You might think I would be hateful or spiteful because of my cards dealt in life. Did I turn away from God when I got sick? No I actually found what <u>you</u> might call "God." For me it is just something I do not understand even with all my scientific knowledge.

What is God for me? God is something I thank every morning I wake up. In my head I say thank you for giving me one more day to see my husband's face, to see my son smile. When I have a good day, I say thank you for letting me breathe easier today than yesterday. When I am sick I say thank you for not taking my life tonight.

At the hospital the other day they had a table set up to register for some running event to help raise money for people with some illness or another. A woman came up and made a big deal about wanting to sign up and help. After making a big deal in front of her friends, she asked what day it was on. It was going to be held on a Sunday. Oh but then she couldn't be there, because she must be at church. What a ridiculous woman. This is very common and my husband and I hear this same silly spout all too much. Please explain to me (because God KNOWS I am not an expert): does Jesus really want your shiny lily white ass sitting on a bench singing some dumb ass song over a hundred years old, impressing really "God" only knows whom rather than helping people in need?

I feel ashamed and sorry for women and men like this. They obviously are ignorant of what their religion is based on. They are walking around with their eyes shuts and are truly unable to see the light. I suppose this is just like bad manners, but sometimes people need a swift kick in the crotch. According to her beliefs she will be weighed on the poor choices she made. Sorry, thanks for playing ma'am, better pick out a pretty new bikini, it's gonna be hot as hell where you are going.

God is not in a book some human wrote down. God is not one religion or another. <u>God Is</u>. Stop blaming God for everything in your life or using God as an excuse. And just maybe once say "thank you for letting me see the sun rise one more morning". Maybe then you too can walk into the light with your eyes wide open.

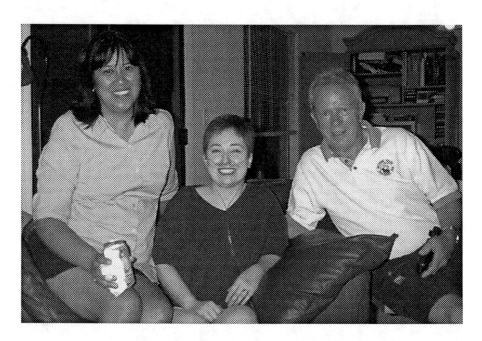

Meg, Carrie and Steve

IV INSPIRING STORIES

In the process of writing this book, I became aware of numerous individuals who had inspiring stories to tell. Each of these stories reveals one or more of the six "elements of healing" discussed in this book. Love is the most central force in each of these stories but it is also clear that there are other elements that have an impact on healing.

Not each of these persons had ARDS, but each of them dealt with a critical – and sometimes fatal – illness. We start with Eric Gebelein, who died while this book was being written.

Eric Gebelein (5-5-46 to 2-3-02)
"Wilderness As Healer"

The story of Eric Gebelein is especially important to me. Eric was a PhD Psychologist whom I knew as a close personal friend and mountain runner. I paced him for the last 22 miles of the Western States' 100-mile foot race in 1982 and he introduced my wife, Lynn, to ultra-marathoning.

Before his death from cancer at age 55, Eric published a wonderful book entitled, "Wilderness As Healer". This book relates Eric's experience with the therapeutic benefits of returning to nature with camping, hiking and living in wilderness settings.

Pets were also very important to Eric, particularly as he faced his cancer foe. In his preface, Eric writes,

> *"The population of our household is pets - 3, humans - 2. The cats are Bubs and Matilda. The dog is Onyx, a black Labrador Retriever.*
> *When I've been in cancer treatment either with post surgical recovery, chemotherapy or radiation, the animals never left my side - they seemed to "know" that something was up and that I was feeling like refried owl poop.*
> *For cancer patients, other aspects of our lives may take a back seat due to the worry and anxiety that cancer commands. Our pets break up the constant attention we can devote to the uncertainty of having cancer and the worry over the outcome. Pets get us outside*

of ourselves and the preoccupation with worry and anxiety around cancer.

Getting a dog was the best thing we ever did! Living with a Labrador Retriever mandates exercise every day (a tired Lab is a happy Lab and their owner is happy, too). I get exercise everyday, which I'm not sure I would have done had I not gotten the dog. On days that I don't feel particularly well, I suppose it would be easy not to go out and go for a walk. But Onyx soon demands it and I do feel better once I'm out in the fresh air, walking by the river, seeing the wildflowers and noticing the animal prints since yesterday. In short, I feel better just for going for a walk with Onyx out in the mountain. I don't have to think about that damned cancer anymore than necessary - it is helpful to give this disease less power."

Eric's book establishes wilderness experiences as healing for many conditions including his own cancer. He outlived his cancer prognosis by many years and states,

"In my opinion, leaving the city was and is the single most important thing we did in battling this disease..."

Though weakened by cancer, Eric continued his wilderness walks with Onyx, his Black Labrador buddy, which his wife, Rebecca, wisely brought into his life. Onyx gave Eric love and got him outside for walks until shortly before his death. Eric writes,

"The usual assortment of blue jays and chipmunks shared the river, the forest and the quiet. It's not like it used to be — hiking, climbing and running up the mountain trails, but it isn't so bad. As far as quality of life...I don't think this could be any better, after all."

Eric passed to the next unknown wilderness on February 3, 2002. His wife, Rebecca and - of course - his dog, Onyx, were joined by about 40 of Eric's friends and family at his home in the woods of the Icicle Valley in Leavenworth, Washington, to celebrate his life and to bury his ashes at the roots of an evergreen tree planted in the memory of this remarkable man.

Eric Gebelein's story reminds us of the healing power of nature, and of pets and love, as we deal with any critical illness.

Sheridan Alonzo
A Memorial: Cherish Your Children

ARDS can strike anyone. In spite of good health and lots of love and prayer, persons afflicted with ARDS may still not survive.

Sheridan Alonzo, 29-year-old Vail ski instructor, mother of two, was admitted with flu-like symptoms, which turned into pneumonia and ARDS. In spite of incredible family support from her husband Dave, her mother Mary, family in Vermont and many friends, she died after a brief hospital stay.

Laura Andersen, a close high school friend, writes:

> *"Sheridan, a class leader and beauty, took me - a nerd - under her wing and instilled self-confidence in me through an honest and unconditional friendship. I always loved her for that. She leaves quite a legacy for her children. Her sudden and unexpected death reminds other mothers to cherish every day with their children - no matter how difficult and tedious it might be. Cherish the opportunity to give your children unconditional love and security."*

The spirit of Sheridan lives on in her children and all those her loved her.

Kathy Larson
ARDS, A Little Known Killer, Can Strike Anyone

Kathy is a writer and one of the members of the NASN – Northwest ARDS Support Network. A healthy 53 year old, she caught a "Y2K bug" and crashed with pneumonia on New Years Eve, 1999. After a battle with ARDS for nearly 2 months, she was discharged. She subsequently published a pamphlet entitled "How To Be A Successful Care Giver".

In the Spring of 2002, Meg Tapucol-Provo hosted a dinner for Northwest ARDS survivors. An incredible thought came to Kathy's mind:

> *"I'm sitting in a room full of dead people. Once dead and now resurrected. What an incredible Easter Story!"*

Kathy continues her recollection:

> *I looked at the smiling faces of five ARDS survivors. I was number six. Half of the people in the room had either died, or been in that place that is between life and death. In Meg's cozy living room, we shared our near-death experiences. Spouses held our hands as the incredible stories unfolded.*
>
> *One young man recounted, "I died at home of a drug overdose, but was resuscitated and taken to a hospital by ambulance. When I died again, they managed to revive me a second time. The third time I passed on, the doctor marked my body for organ harvesting with a felt pen and left me in "the cold room. My best friend had heard of my illness and hurried to the hospital. A nurse informed him of my demise. Insisting on the opportunity of saying goodbye to me, he was taken to my room, where he noticed that my leg moved!"*
>
> *The now-very-alive young man continues his story stating what the nurse said next: "Some leg movement is normal right after death." The multi-resurrected young man laughs as he relates that after one more twitch of his foot the nurse was called to "Check the corpse." Detecting a pulse, the nurse sent for a doctor. "I was back for the third time." His wife*

just shakes her head.

While dead, or between worlds, many of our journeys were terrible and painful to share. Most of us eventually came to a place of incredible joy, love and peace. Many of us feel that we have been sent back to do something important, but not sure just what that might be.

ARDS and other life threatening illnesses cause us to rethink the meaning and purpose of life. Kathy continues her comments on ARDS:

ARDS can strike anyone - infant to elderly, rich or poor, healthy or sick There is no cure. The only hope for the victim is to be placed on a ventilator, under strict supervision, until the lungs decide whether or not to repair themselves. Prayer and loving support seem to be the best medicines. There are numerous ways that the syndrome can be triggered.

I had contracted pneumonia, another woman had a Caesarian section, a male doctor had fallen from a ski-lift chair, and a young man had been in a car accident. A woman, now in her twenties, had drowned when she was eight, having been at the bottom of a lake for twelve minutes. Our Intensive Care and Rehabilitation Hospital stays ranged from two to nine months and the combined hospital bills totaled in the millions of dollars. Most of us are dealing with the fall-out of the ARDS. Memory loss, nerve damage, shortness of breath, and fear of another illness to haunt us to one degree or another.

In spite of the disabilities suffered by Kathy and other ARDS patients, they have continued to be active and to enjoy life. Rather than dwelling on the past, they are living in the present and planning for the future.

Jeff Nicholson
Remarkable Artwork - - By A Quadriplegic

One of the most meaningful visits during my recovery from ARDS was from Jeff Nicholson, a 41 year old quadriplegic due to a major automobile accident at age 22. Jeff is the son of my longtime medical transcriptionist, LeeAnna Nicholson. Jeff reminded me that "where there is a will, there is a way." I felt that if Jeff could be so productive with his disabilities, then I, too, could return to a productive life as a physician in spite of any residual limitations I might have.

Jeff found his artistic ability making illustrations by holding a pencil with his teeth. He recently has advanced from black and white to color illustrations and hopes someday to hold an art show. I visualize joining him in speaking engagements about dealing with life crisis and disabilities.

Examples such as the artwork shown required over 200 hours of meticulous work and can be purchased by writing Jeff at jeffreybob@webtv.net.

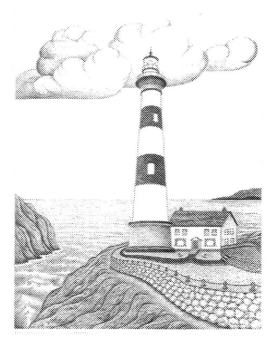

Guiding Light
This black-and-white illustration of a lighthouse, when viewed through a magnifying glass is amazing in its detail.

David Ross
"Diving Under the Waves"

David Ross's first visit to Hawaii taught him one of the lasting lessons of his life. Although he did not have ARDS or other life threatening illness, his story of riding the waves contains lessons for each of us.

> *Always I had been entranced by the breathtaking scenery of the coastlines of Hawaii, and now was my chance to actually enter those beautiful waters. The waves were breaking unusually high that day, and I was prepared to "ride the waves" and enjoy our family time at the beach. After assuring my wife and three children that I knew what I was doing, I proceeded to walk upright into the wave to ride it back in. Instead, I was turned head over heels, completely disoriented, out of breath and ready to give up on those waves. Then the friend who picked me up out of the sand said, "David, what you should do is dive under the wave, then come up on the other side of it and you can easily ride it in." I tried it, and it worked beautifully. No more crashes or accidents, just gently resting as the wave carried me to shore.*

> *Since then I have learned to "dive under" in a lot of life's circumstances. Because a lot of our ministry is done cross-culturally, in other nations, I have learned that the proper way to "enter a new culture" is to dive under - taking all the gifts, plans, ideas, even financial assistance or other good things we may want to do for the people of that culture - and just remain there, under the waves, until those people themselves lift me up and are ready to receive.*

This experience has made David a learner as well as a teacher and a receiver as well as a giver of himself. David concludes:

> *Since that memorable time I have practiced "diving under" in many different situations - letting go of control, letting God and sometimes other people direct and heal, provide and protect me in ways I could never do myself.*

David has a website for his ministry - www.ywam-aiim.org.

Dee Storey
Music, Touch, and Humor

Dee Storey is an ARDS survivor who went into the hospital April 14, 2000 and was discharged May 12, 2000. In her pulmonary rehabilitation, she was on 3 liters of oxygen about 20 hours a day. She writes how music, touch and humor were important elements in her healing.

Music

A friend had brought in my CD player and my favorite music. I listened to the Stone Poneys (with early Linda Ronstadt), James Taylor, Mozart, The Beatles, and Dixie Chicks – an odd assortment. Well many of my nurses had never heard of The Stone Poneys or James Taylor. WHEW! I'm only 50 and when I was on the vent, these singers seemed so lively and so honoring of my youth and happier days. One day a young nurse was going through the CDs and found the Fly album by the Dixie Chicks and we all toe tapped to the song about Earl having to die. How much we laughed. Okay, I had a vent in my mouth, but my spirits soared. I smiled from within. When I got home from the hospital and saw the video, my caregiver and I laughed and laughed. Thank you Dixie Chicks.

Touch

I was going nuts about having awful hair. It had been covered with all sorts of tape from the vent and generally been a tangled mess. After I got off the vent, I wanted the nurses to shave my head. They said "NO". So I begged and pleaded, in writing as I didn't have a speaking voice. They agreed to allow my hairdresser, Lynn, to come in CCU and cut my hair....IF I could sit up in a chair. I was inspired. I don't know how long it took me to get from lying down to sitting up, but I had a big smile for Lynn when she made a hospital call. She cut my hair and made me promise not to tell anyone who did "the do" because the back looked ragged because I suddenly ran out of steam and had to get flat in bed. She made me smile then and I'm smiling as I write this. She walked in CCU and brought in the smells of a salon...smells that I never thought I'd experience again. She made it all seem like an adventure. I smiled later when I wondered about the many rules that must have been broken to allow Lynn in CCU...sometimes rules are made to be broken.

A couple of days after I got my hair cut, I wanted it washed. Betty, the licensed practical nurse, knew all about using "real water" when washing someone's hair when they were in bed. "Real water?" I asked. "Real water," she promised. Well, Betty tilted my bed way back until I was sure I would slide out of bed on my head. Then she encased my head in a lawn size garbage bag and she began to use water and soap to create such an experience! Betty's side of the bed was perfectly dry. The other side of the bed was sopping wet. What a hoot! We all giggled. We all clapped our hands. We laughed about it for days and days. I didn't fall out of bed from the hair washing, but I often wondered if I was going to fall out of bed laughing about the experience.

Humor

My brother brought in drawings done by my nieces to hang in my CCU room. My 8-year old niece, Taylor, is a very good artist, concentrating on people. My 6-year old niece, Maddie, is a very good artist who just happens to have a very creative approach to life and artistic interpretation. When I awoke from my drug-induced haze, I looked at Maddie's picture and thought I saw something that was phallic. I thought it was the drugs that made me misinterpret what she had drawn and written. Visitors would come in and talk about Maddie's picture in a very round about manner and giggle. Nurses talked about Maddie's picture in a round about manner and giggled. When I got out of the hospital, I called Maddie and told her that I thought she was a good artist. She said "of course." I asked her what the picture was about and she said, "My bunny." YIKES! I was amazed. Her father was amazed. My friends were amazed. We never would have gathered that she had drawn a toy bunny. We all thought that she had drawn something not quite so innocent. I still have that picture on my wall at home.

Visitors still giggle when they see this picture. I still smile.

Humor is an ironic thing in CCU. There's not much going on that's funny. In spite of everything, my nurses kept things hoppin' and happin'. Dee is still 'hoppin' and actively involved in national programs related to ARDS.

Katherine Blaydes
A "Three Month Nap"

This is an email sent to me by a nurse (RN) showing the complexity of ARDS – with a favorable outcome. In spite of the technical terms, the message should be clear to everyone.

> *I am an ARDS survivor. I was diagnosed in July of 1997, following a bacterial pneumonia at the age of 34. At the time of my illness I had been working in the ICU as an RN for 12 years.*
>
> *During my course with ARDS I had seven chest tubes - the result of barotrauma from the Jet vent. I was trached and on a vent for 3 months. I went into DIC. I developed hepatic and renal failure (MultiSystems organ failure), developed hypotensive shock, and was on Dopamine for an extended period.*
>
> *On August 17, 1997, my heart rate dropped into the teens and ended with a cardiac arrest, obviously with successful resuscitation efforts. A week following the cardiac arrest the doctors started to bring me up from the drug-induced coma. They wanted me to help them fight it out if I could. It worked.*
>
> *I remember trying to tell my family I could hear them and I could "see" them with me. I have a clear memory of only one day - August 17, the day I "crashed". I can remember clearly the lady who did our dry cleaning coming to see me in ICU - she is Muslim. I was laughing at the ICU nurses who were trying to throw her out because she was kneeling and praying in Arabic.*
>
> *I remember the nurses talking about how sad it was that I was only 34 and was "leaving" my family. They were talking about the charge nurse going home early because she didn't want to be there when I coded. I remember Father Patrick coming into the room giving me Last Rites. I remember thinking I must have been in a very bad plane crash. (I had flown a few days before I became ill and the last memory I have before waking up in ICU is flying home. I was awake and alert for the first 3 days of my admission, but I can't remember that at all).*
>
> *During my recovery my family and friends talked to me*

about what had been going on while I took my "3 month nap". They would joke with me about my hair being a mess and it was like I had walked on the moon the first day when I could brush my teeth without help. I drove the nurses in ICU insane. I fussed about the A-Line and the Swan. I hated the vent and the trach. I wouldn't let an RN suction me (they are horrible at that) only RT could come near me with the suction. I would lean over the bed trying to see if the chest tubes were draining - not an easy task with 4 on the left and 3 on the right. I had one RT who would stand there and cry trying to wean me. She could make me breathe telling me she wasn't going to allow me to be vent dependent even if it killed both of us. My husband, God love him - would cry watching me trying to hold a spoon and I couldn't do it. But he wouldn't do it for me: he made me do it. We called everyone we knew the first day I could cut my own nails with the clippers. For almost 5 months after my discharge I didn't have enough strength to work the clippers. The recovery was hard. It took me a full year to come back to what I would consider almost normal. I didn't suffer any of the PTSD that people talk about really. But I came away with a sense of peace. I know there is something beyond this and even though the body may die, who we are never does. The NDE (near death experience) is, as they say, "a whole nuther story." (laughing)

Katherine's story gives witness to the powers of love, prayer, touch and humor in her long battle with ARDS.

Christiane Solbach
ARDS Is An International Disease

This message from Christiane Solbach in Germany shows that ARDS is international as are advanced treatment methods like "ECMO" – Extra-Corporeal Membrane Oxygenation. Along with high-tech treatments, touch and love remain important elements of healing, as shown in the following email:

> *I survived ARDS in 1995 after a Legionnaire's infection. I was treated with the help of the ECMO and was in a drug-induced coma for five weeks. I have very vivid memories of this time and most of them are terrible.*
>
> *What is interesting is that my parents helped me a great deal simply by being there. When my mother caressed my arm, for example, the fever went down a few degrees. I also moved around and kicked a lot. They couldn't keep me calm- not even with plenty of medication. But when my parents came into the ICU — I stopped kicking and thrashing.*
>
> *When I was in the ICU, right after the ECMO, I found out that I was not alone. I was sharing a room with Eldeltraut, a woman of about my age. She developed ARDS when she had chickenpox and was flown into the clinic that I was and was also on the ECMO. We shared the same fate and stayed together for five weeks. We couldn't talk because of the tube (Trachea) but we had eye-contact. You can't imagine what it meant for us. If one was feeling depressed and sad, the other tried to cheer up. (We wrote little letters to each other that the nurses had to pass on.) It was like the turbo-booster of motivation for us. We tried to fight the sickness together! After a while, the doctors and nurses called us the "siamese twins". We developed such a strength together that it must have been very difficult for the nurses at times. One would fight for the other... My parents came daily to the hospital at the time to visit me and adopted Edeltraut as well since she was so far from her home that she didn't have many visitors. It was amazing, but we managed to be transferred to our "home hospitals" on the same date. One of our doctors stated, "the 31st of August is*

your birthday from now on, because you both have survived something very difficult". Exactly one year afterwards, Edeltraut and I went back to the clinic and walked into the ICU to celebrate our first birthday with the whole staff of the ICU. Now, that's what I call a party!!! In my mind and soul she is my sister and always will be. We don't see much of each other because we live far apart but we talk very frequently on the phone. We share something that will always be a special bond between us.

Christiane's email message relates to support from love and prayer:

I think that it not only takes machines and medical treatment for a patient to recover. The patient has to be a fighter and needs a reason to survive. That's where relatives and friends come in. I was told afterwards of all the people that prayed for me during that time, people that didn't even know me and people of Christian, Jewish and Muslim background. That gave me immense strength during the coma because I felt that I was loved and that people sent me strength to keep on fighting.

My nephew was always by my side when it became difficult for me. At the time he was ten years old and he was so positively sure that I would survive. I always had a very deep relationship with him, and he, as well as my parents, were the reason for me to live. I am sure you understand that. I "saw" my parents during the coma while the doctor told them that only their love for me could heal me. That was the "turbo booster" for me!

Christiane relates how ARDS changed her:

Since I had the ARDS a lot of things changed for me. I became a different person (I would say) because of my near death experiences and the time that I had to think my life over. Before I got sick I flew around as a flight attendant and led a fairly superficial life. Now I am no longer restless and have finally found my inner peace. I also found true love in my parents and my husband.

GOD not only gave me my life back, but He granted me a better one....

Music also has meaning for Christane Solbach:

> *I have a music CD that is very precious to me. It is relaxation music and very soothing. I feel down or tired, I put it on. I relax automatically now just listening to it. All the time I wondered why and I finally found the answer. My breathing adjusts automatically to the rhythm of the music and gives me peace and quiet. Every time I have trouble breathing I get panic attacks. I thought that I would never "learn" to breathe again and the doctors and nurses didn't reassure me much. Well, the music is like a crutch for me now. I listen to it and I can relax.*

Since her ARDS, Christiane has revisited her hospital for a symposium and banquet in honor of the Chief of the Medical Department. She joined three other survivors who exchanged experiences with each other. They shared the conviction that anybody who survives ARDS is a fighter and can be proud of their accomplishment.

Sheri Martin – Do You Believe In Angels?

Sheri Martin tells a story where attentive love, prayer and belief led to a miraculous recovery. And do you believe in Angels? … and doctors?

Sheri starts her story with how she developed ARDS:

> *On March 26, 1997 I went to the hospital to have a partial hysterectomy. Everything went really well. I remember developing a severe cough and lower back pain. That was the time when the comet was visible in the sky for quite a while. I remember my husband walking me across the hall into another room to see it. I wanted so badly to see it. I couldn't make it to the window. I was totally exhausted and out of breath. I suppose everyone thought it was from the surgery. I had my surgery on a Wednesday morning. On Friday I called my husband at work to tell him that I was really sick. He was out on calls that morning. I just wanted him to know how sick I felt.*
>
> *On Saturday I was getting worse. When the nurse came in and checked my oxygen level it was so low that she thought the machine was broken. They brought in another machine. It showed that my oxygen was too low. They moved me to I.C.U. that evening and put me on oxygen. That night my husband and family went home thinking the doctor would just give me some antibiotics and in the morning I would be better. The last awake moment I remember, the Doctor and Nurse were telling me I was very sick and needed to be on a ventilator. I was so scared. I knew inside that I was dying. My nurse was so wonderful. She said the sinner's prayer with me. I was a Christian, but was not living for the Lord at that time. I was afraid I was going to die.*
>
> *When my husband got to the hospital they were putting me on the ventilator. I had signed all of the papers myself. The Doctor was looking at the x-rays of my lungs. "Only partial lungs," the Doctor told my husband, Ernie, "she's dying and we're doing all we can to save her." Ernie quickly got out of his way! The doctors told my family that I probably wouldn't make it through the night. My best friend, Cathy, came in from Arkansas and stayed all night in my room praying for me.*

During the night a man came into my room and asked Cathy if he could pray for me. He did and then left. No one ever saw him again. She thinks he was an angel. Well I lasted through the night.

The hospital let family stay in the room all of the time except during shift changes, early in the morning, and then in the evening. There was a lot of prayer going up for me, but my condition stayed the same. The doctors expected me to die. My husband kept telling them that God was going to heal me. They had Christian television on 24 hours a day in my room.

On my 8th day on the ventilator my husband and daughter were in my room and the doctor told my husband that I had made a little progress, and that I may be off the vent in about a month. Ernie spoke to our daughter and said, "Shelby, we need to just start thanking and praising God for healing your mom. Even thought we are not seeing any progress, we still need to thank Him in advance." So they were praying and thanking God for healing my body and letting me live. They looked over at me and I was moving all over the bed. My husband thought I was having a seizure! Shelby looked up at the TV and saw a woman singing and dancing to the Lord. She looked over at me and I was keeping time with her! I was dancing with her. I was in a drug-induced coma.

My husband went home that night knowing that the Lord had healed my body. The next morning Ernie was back up at the hospital bright and early. When the Doctor came in Ernie told him he didn't need to look at my charts, he just needed to take me off of life support. My Doctor thought Ernie had lost his mind, but when he walked in and asked me how I was, I gave him a thumbs-up sign. He ordered an X-ray immediately. He couldn't believe it! I was off life support within 4 hours!

They took me off of the ventilator on a Monday. All week I told everyone I was going home. They said I was too sick. Well, on Saturday I went home! My lung doctor didn't even want to see me again. I think it was too weird for him! I never went to any of the doctors after that!

*But all of that is behind me now. I have never written down my story before. I hope it will help people to know, **Don't***

Give Up!

Others have spoken of "angels" as does Sheri, but I must say I have no direct experience in that regard. I am aware that "doctors" are real – but not always right! However, modern medicine continues to advance and the mortality rate for ARDS patients is going down. In spite of the advances in medicine, it is important to remember those elements of healing which are "beyond medicine".

Jack Yonts
Wisconsin Pastor Is A Living Miracle

(Based on local news article by Claire Mangin, Post-Crescent correspondent, Fox Cities, Wisconsin, with permission and also with permission of Jack Yonts. Original article, 9-9-00)

Here is an inspiring story supporting the power of prayer, personal faith and determination. This is an example of a "return from the hopeless". Once again it is shown that we doctors don't know it all nor have a perfect record in predicting outcome. Jack's recovery after declining a lung transplant procedure was truly a miracle, which is to say, beyond outside current medical understanding. At the same time we are, once again, challenged to consider Love, Faith, Positive Attitude and Prayer as "Elements of Healing".

Don't tell the Rev. Jack Yonts that stories about miracles are found only in the Bible. Yonts stared down death more than once during his ordeal with ARDS. He and his family were told that up to 70% of ARDS victims die within a few days.

"Jack Yonts" is no doubt a miracle. He would have had better odds at winning the lottery," said Dr. Michael Maguire of Fox Valley Pulmonary Medicine in Wisconsin. "I can count maybe three or four miracles during my years of practice, but this definitely tops the list. When we had nothing more to offer him, their prayers took over".

A "Cold" Leads To ARDS

The ARDS couldn't have come at a worse time. Yonts and his wife, Lori, had just brought home their adopted infant daughter, Lily. Five weeks later he thought he had a cold and went to bed early. At 2 a.m. he awoke and found he couldn't breathe. Since he was still fighting to breathe the next morning, his wife took him to the local hospital. He was diagnosed as having bronchitis with pneumonia and sent home with antibiotics. But his condition deteriorated and "We were getting scared", Lori said. He was admitted to the hospital. "I really felt like I was going to die that night. I just couldn't get any air," Jack said.

In the ICU he was put on a ventilator and the last thing he remembers, before being placed in a drug-induced coma, is his favorite song, 'Can't Nobody Do Me Like Jesus'. Even on the ventilator he was purple from the waist up and had very low blood oxygen levels. Doctors told the family that he would most likely die before day's end.

Prayer Power

"There is nothing more we can do but pray", said Jack' s father, also a minister. The family and friends went to the hospital chapel and prayed for the next one-to-two hours. Dan Sharp, Jack's assistant pastor, visited Jack daily and on Easter Sunday was told Jack probably would not make it through the day. Dan went straight to the church, informed everyone of Jack's condition, cancelled the regular Easter service, and called a prayer meeting. Later that day, Dan returned to the hospital and found Jack's color had returned to normal.

More Complications

Over the next eight weeks, Jack had 14 pneumothoraxes (holes blown in the lungs from the ventilator pressure) requiring chest tubes to reinflate the lungs. He had multiple organ failure, with kidney, liver and heart dysfunction, compounded by pulmonary emboli (clots traveling to the lungs). The family was told that each of these problems made the prognosis about 10% worse and, "We have nothing more to offer him".

As the prayers of many continued, Jack Yonts, the "hopeless case", once again stunned the doctors by stabilizing. A team of experts said, "A lung transplant is the only option left." The family and Jack were told he would be flown to the University Hospital in Madison for the transplant. They were also told that he would require medicines costing up to $1,200 a month; he could not drink tap water; he must avoid crowds including church services and he would have a life expectancy of five to six years.

A Critical Decision

Yonts and his family prayed together and made a decision: "Either God is going to heal me or I am going to die", Jack said. They turned away the transplant team who all thought we were "nuts".

It was on that day that Jack's condition turned around. He had not been able to sit up or eat but he could within 5 days and was moved out of the ICU. He began lifting weights and dangling his legs. After 2 weeks he begged to be out of bed to walk. He was allowed to walk with help to the door, as far as the ventilator tube would allow.

Headed Home

Jack's pleas to be taken off the ventilator were rejected until a weekend doctor decided to show him he couldn't breathe without it. Jack did so well he was never hooked up to the ventilator again. Feeling confident, Jack announced that he would be home in 4 weeks to celebrate his 13th wedding anniversary. Three weeks later his tracheotomy tube was removed and Jack could speak for the first time, his first words being an enthusiastic, "Thank you, Jesus!" Seven days later, as predicted, Jack was discharged to go home where the family had an anniversary dinner delivered from their favorite restaurant.

"It is incredible to be home after my 3-month ordeal and now I'm back in my own house and own bed, at home with my lovely wife and little girl," Jack expressed. He concluded by saying, "This whole thing has been a great faith-building experience, and has caused me to have a greater belief in the miraculous".

Readers may be interested in reading the book, "With Every Breath I Praise Him! – The Miraculous Healing of Jack E. Yonts II," as told to Jim H. Yohe. For information, contact Jack E. Yonts II, P. O. Box 2533, Appleton, WI 54912.

Jeanie Knecht – Dogs Defeat Death

Jeanie Knecht is another "miracle" survivor who tells her story quite briefly:

> *I'm 49 years old, and I live in Vancouver, Washington (the Portland metro area). I have two 12 year-old dogs that are Doberman mix.*
>
> *I don't remember the night, but in January I went to the Urgent care for nausea and then went into shock and went into a coma for three and a half weeks. I was in the hospital for five weeks. Then every organ shut down except for my liver and my brain. I had a pacemaker, blood transfusion, was on a ventilator for a month, dialysis because my kidneys failed, pneumonia, and acute respiratory failure.*
>
> *They said I was going to die, so all my brothers and sisters came out and they called a priest and now they're all religious again. I could hear the priest and I was really mad because I had no intention of dying and I thought they were all giving up on me. I could hear people talking. People shouldn't say things in front of a patient in a coma.*
>
> *I wanted to take a long, long rest, but no one was mentioning my dogs, and I got so worried about them and heard dogs barking. I didn't know if I had been in an auto accident and they had been with me or what happened. I decided I had to wake up to find out about them, so I made the hugest effort I've ever made, and threw myself back, and I woke up. I don't know what happened.*

Amnesia is a very common occurance with ARDS. In my own case, I have no memory of the events leading to my ARDS or for about two months after my accident. Although actual memories may be blocked, the person with ARDS continues to receive healing input from love, prayer, touch, humor, music and pets.

Shannon Kalisher
The Magic Of Music – And Brothers

Shannon was a 29 year old Research Assistant living in Boulder, Colorado, when she contracted ARDS. She tells this moving story about the power of music and brotherly love:

My illness began as Strep Throat which progressed to pneumonia. I then developed sepsis as the bacteria moved into my blood stream. Gradually all of my organs failed and I was diagnosed with ARDS. Throughout my hospital stay I required 10 chest tubes, a trach tube, feeding tube, and eventually part of my left lung was removed.

I still deal with some after-effects of ARDS - shortness of breath, decreased lung capacity, a chronic cough, vascular issues and the emotional trauma, but the worst is definitely behind me. I spent 3 1/2 months in Boulder Community Hospital under the care of some of the most amazing nurses, doctors, respiratory therapists, physical therapists, Xray technicians, music therapists, janitorial staff and volunteers. I know that I wouldn't be here without their love, support, wisdom and expertise.

Nothing could protect my little brother, Patrick, from the pain of seeing me, his oldest sister, critically ill in the Intensive Care Unit. There I was on a ventilator, with a feeding tube, 10 chest tubes, and a trach tube keeping me alive.

I can't imagine what it must have felt like to walk into that room and see someone you love in that state. But when Patrick was physically present with me, it was like he never left. He was my little brother, the one I nurtured and took care of when we were young. During this time however, he was the one who held me up.

There is one day in particular that stands out in my mind as a time that he truly saved me by being there. The hospital in which I stayed had a music therapist, Willow, who provided various services for the patients. Willow explained to me that during a session she would bring her guitar or keyboard. Normally she would sing some songs and then I would have an opportunity to write my own thoughts on paper, (I could not speak at this time because of my trach tube) and then she would put my words to music. I was initially disinterested by the idea of these sessions. It was all I could do to stay awake with all of the pain medication that was pumping through my frail body and I was reluctant to interact with anyone besides my family and my favorite doctors and nurses.

One evening Patrick came to visit me and we had some rare time to ourselves. Willow entered my room during our visit and asked if I would like to write a song with her. She held her guitar in her arms and her eyes struck me as being very safe and sincere - maybe it wouldn't be so bad, I thought. I agreed to the session but I asked Patrick to stay with me.

Willow turned the florescent lights off in my room and turned on a soft lamp instead. There were no candles that evening, but when I think of that time with Willow and my brother, I can't help but think that there was a presence of fire, warmth and light around us all.

Willow gave me a pad of paper and instructed me to "just write anything that came to my mind". Feeling apprehensive, I just layed there for a bit wondering what I was "supposed to write" in my notebook. My brother sat by my side running his fingers through my hair and listening to Willow play her soft music. I wasn't feeling particularly creative or eloquent that evening in my sterile hospital bed, but then the tears came rolling down my cheeks like a pebble down a steep mountain. I put my pencil on the paper and I remember just writing - writing what now reads as disjointed, random thoughts on a white sheet of paper but at the time, these words served as my first release of the deep emotions I had been feeling for weeks. I realized that I needed to get this out - I needed to write "my song". The tears continued to fall as the thoughts spilled out of my broken mind and heart.

When I finished, I handed the scribbles to Willow and she began to play a few simple chords on her guitar, softly singing my jumbled lyrics without judgment. I began to sing with her in my mind and my brother, so strong and scared held my hand and silently cried. His head fell in my lap and my clean white sheet absorbed his tears. I knew that he felt the intensity of my words and my message of pain and confusion. The lyrics expressed my need to know why this was happening to me, how this all happened and what was going to happen next. The fear and anxiety that swept my body each day in the hospital came out on my piece of paper that night.

I thank Willow for providing me with a channel for expressing my thoughts. In retrospect, that session definitely served as a vehicle for me to realize the fervor of emotions that accompanied me during my stay in the hospital. One cannot go through an illness like ARDS and not be overcome by the feelings of anger, confusion, anxiety and fear on some level. I continued my music sessions with Willow for the remainder of my stay. My "songs" became a little more coherent and clear as my mind recovered from the trauma of the illness and eventually I was able to sing my own lyrics with my own voice.

When I finally got to go home after 3 1/2 months in the hospital, I continued to write "my songs". It helped me so much to get the painful thoughts out of my head and onto paper. Some of the "songs" are a collection of random memories that have haunted me in my sleep while others are tributes to the many individuals who played such integral parts in my survival and ultimate recovery from this devastating illness.

Shannon's example of music therapy is the most interesting I have encountered in my studies. Creating a song with lyrics related to the patient's emotions is a fantastic idea. Hopefully other musicians will follow this lead as in Shannon's story.

Michael 'Anvil' Weglin
Suicide, ARDS and New Life

Mike's story can be read at his website:
www.anvilmedia.net/assc

Mike's ARDS began with aspiration during CPR when he nearly died following an intentional suicidal overdose of a variety of drugs including codeine, Prozac, Darvocet, Benadryl, beta blocker, and tranquilizers. His memory of vivid dreams is well described, as it has been by other ARDS victims.

It almost seems like a dream to me when Michael visited me in my Rehab room at Harborview Hospital. I vividly remember his broad smile, optimistic outlook, and loving manner - but most of all I remember the button-down shirt and tie signifying the use of his fingers for a skill I still lacked. He assured me that skill would return.

When I asked if there was anything he lost from his ARDS ordeal, he responded without delay, "My libido." This was reassuring since I, too, felt an absence of sex drive. Mike's account of his experience with visiting me and with his own libido story is worth reading in his website.

Mike is now married and working to help others design websites. Interestingly, he has taken up skydiving and sells his service doing video recording of others doing sky dives. No, I don't think this is crazy or suicidal. It just reflects Mike's intent to get the most out of life. After all, when you've already come back more than once from the jaws of death, what have you got to lose? A number of persons over age 80 have done skydiving so maybe I'm missing something. It sounds safer than riding a motorcycle … or riding in a ski chairlift!

Sue Hart
For Everything There Is A Season (Ecclesiastes 3: 1-8)

This is a remarkable story of a 40-year-old single mother who has dealt with an undiagnosed disease with features of multiple sclerosis, fibromyalgia, and other ailments. The description of her discomfort, inconclusive diagnostic studies, and her own personal commitment to healing and wellness is inspirational to all of us. Here is her story as she tells it.

It was a dark, rainy Friday the 13th in November 1998. My daughter, Jennifer, and I were driving home from the store when we were in an accident. Not much damage was done to the car, but the physical damage to me was significant but slow to reveal itself.

Within four days I was at the doctors for the first of many appointments. For the first year my problems stayed in my left arm and neck area. After a couple months I saw a neurologist but by then the insurance company had their own doctor evaluate me. They said I should be cured and discontinued benefits.

A Time to Suffer:

Thirteen months after the accident they thought that surgery on the nerve at the left wrist would help some of the pain I was having. The day before surgery it was canceled for insurance reasons. While I was upset at this, it was the first of many blessings. I soon learned that in every disappointment there is a blessing. The more I let go and stopped trying to make things happen, the easier it was for me.

January 2000, fourteen months after the accident, I was tucking in my shirt while getting ready for work and I heard a loud pop. I could not straighten up and my legs were going numb. I went to the doctor and he put me in a neck brace, ordered more physical therapy, traction and medications. My team of doctors consisted of the neurosurgeon, a new neurologist, a pain specialist, a pain psychologist and of course the doctors who did the tests. I do believe they were all doing their best to help me, but I continued to worsen.

My right side started going numb. By the end of July my face and tongue were numb. The doctors were baffled. August brought more tests to see if I had a brain tumor or signs of MS. They tested me for Diabetes, Parkinson's, Lyme Disease and more.

By September, 2000 the pain became so intense I did not want to venture far from home for fear of having one of the attacks that would cripple me. I came home from work too tired to cook myself dinner. My speech was slurred. My balance was off and I was having difficulty in walking. My doctor told me to get my final papers in order.

I could not function without pain medication. A day without it left me physically debilitated. I knew that the pain medication only covered up symptoms, and I sought non-drug alternatives such as humor.

A Time to Laugh:

I am a firm believer in the healing power of humor so I made it a point to find a way to make someone laugh everyday. I did this by finding a story from different Internet sites. I found Patch Adams M.D. "GESUNDHEIT!" on tape. He helped me to understand why people were pulling away from me and he reminded me that doctors are human too. His tapes encouraged me and I found new hope.

I read a little bit each night before I went to bed from books like Tuesdays with Morrie, Front Porch Tales, Ecclesiastics, and Corinthians etc. I prayed for strength, courage and the ability to laugh. I changed my perception of my situation and found that the reality was not as bad as I thought. By becoming focused on what I COULD do instead of what I COULD NOT I found freedom from my fears.

A Time to Learn:

While I would never wish for anyone to go through what I have, I know I have an appreciation for life I never would have had without everything that followed that fateful Friday the 13th.

I have learned from my experience that there is a big difference in accepting our limitations vs. using them as an excuse to give up. In acceptance, there is realism. In giving up there is bitterness and blame. I know that each and every one of us has the strength to handle the situations that come our way. We have to first be willing to accept that we can handle the situation, reach deep within ourselves for the strength and then reach out for the encouragement that we need.

I learned to let go and trust that God will handle things in time. With each disappointment I looked for a blessing and if I could not find it I knew it would be revealed to me in time. Amazingly, I found a joy and a peace greater then I could have imagined.

I know that people come and go in our lives. We meet people sometimes only for a moment and will soon be forgotten. Others stay in our hearts for a lifetime. I will always remember... those who encouraged me... my daughters' love... those who showed compassion... my counselor's encouragement... those who gave me hope and those who made me laugh.

I now know that doctors are not God, but human and should be treated with kindness too. I learned that humor is powerful medicine. I learned... the importance of family and friends...the comfort of a pet's unconditional love... the warmth of smiles... the power of compassionate touch... the healing energy of dancing. I learned that some people do not want to heal and that makes me sad.

I learned that how we treat people effects not only their lives, but ours as well. I learned that we can make a difference, if we so choose.

I learned the elements for healing are the same elements as those needed for the quality of life we wish to obtain.

I decided to try to live my life so that I leave those I meet in a positive way. Even if I meet someone for a moment I want to give them the gift of a smile. If they have a minute, I'd like to share a laugh and if they care to linger perhaps we can share a dance.

Although Sue did not have ARDS, her way of dealing with problems is a model for all of us, and to quote Nietsche:

> **"We should consider every day lost on which we have not danced at least once. And we should consider every truth false which was not accompanied by at least one laugh."**

Heather Favale
Triathlete In Spite Of ARDS

Heather's story includes elements of healing- love, prayer and pets (10!), which helped her recover to a high level of fitness – in spite of predictions and PTSD (Post-Traumatic Stress Syndrome)

I am a two-year survivor of ARDS. I am 31 years old and reside in Carbondale, Illinois. I am a health education teacher. My hobbies include swimming, running, and spending quality time with loved ones and my 10 pets (six cats and four dogs).

Not a day goes by that I don't think about my complications with ARDS two years ago. The doctors told my family that I only had a 10% chance of survival. A priest was called in to read me my last rights. I was in a coma for four weeks and on life support for six weeks. With the power of love, prayer, and God, I pulled through. The staff at the hospital, my family, friends, and colleagues all call me the" miracle child".

Having ARDS set me back physically and of course emotionally. I was and still am a very active person. I was told by doctors that I probably would never be able to run again because of the damage done to my lungs. Shortly after my release from the hospital -about four months later - I was running two miles. Eventually, I was able to run four, five, and six miles. One year after my release from the hospital I participated and completed a mini triathlon and nearly beat my time from seven years ago. I am also a Master's swimmer. Although I lost much oxygen capacity from lung damage caused by ARDS, I am a faster and more efficient swimmer now than before my illness.

Up until my diagnoses my family had never heard about ARDS. They were told that most people don't survive. My family spent days researching ARDS on-line and in the library. Now that I know more about ARDS it makes me wonder how I survived.

Breathing is so much different now than I can ever recall before. I can't take deep breaths like I used to. I can feel the weakness from scarring of my lungs. There is always this sense of tightness. This is a constant reminder of my ordeal two years ago.

January 12, 1999 was a horrible day. But each year, January 12th is a celebration of life for me. I remember feeling like I was dying. I remember my last words before I slipped into a coma. I remember the fear and anxiety I experienced. It is easy to use words to describe to people what I remember and what I felt; however, they will never be able to understand the true emotion behind my story.

Currently, I am in therapy to deal with my illness. Two years later it still affects me dearly. Not a day goes by that I don't think about how close I was to death. People ask me "Did you see the light?" My response is, "No, I did not see the light but I did have two dreams in which God asked me if I wanted to live or die." My response to God was "I want life." Living is special. I am a survivor. My spirit is strong. Life goes on.....

Here again is another "miracle child" ... who defied the doctors' gloomy prognosis. For someone who was told she would never be able to run again, to complete a mini-triathlon can be viewed as a miracle.

Courtney Ann Shelstad (5-18-82 to 7-10-99)
Our Gift From God

This memorial was written by Courtney's mother, Colleen, whom I met in Chicago on August 24, 2002 in association with a fund-raising walk event organized by the ARDS Foundation USA (Previously "Illinois"). Colleen was accompanied by her husband, Jim, and sons, Kyle and Chris.

Even though she had just turned seventeen, Courtney was never one to take life for granted. She believed in living everyday as if it were her last. Expressing her love and kindness to everyone she knew, Courtney believed "Smiling is contagious", and "Happiness is a perfume you cannot pour on others without getting a few drops on yourself." This beautiful gift from God was wise beyond her years and she also was an athlete. She took first place overall in the Wisconsin Downhill Jr. Race in 1999 and played Varsity Volleyball her junior. year. When Courtney was as young as four, she had goals, and everyday of her life she would take one step forward to reach those goals. She often stated that she wanted to be a teacher and a pediatrician to find cures for diseases.

At the end of June, 1999, Courtney had just finished her Junior year final exams, had Senior pictures taken, finished taking her ACT tests for college entry and was ready to go with our family for a long weekend to North Carolina over the Fourth of July. On July 1, 1999, it was obvious that Courtney was not feeling well. Even though she had had Mononucleosis in May and was still on antibiotics for a sinus infection, a little nagging dry cough was still there. We called her doctor back home and told her Courtney was complaining of her collarbone burning. The doctor said it must be the mono. When we arrived in North Carolina at 7:00 that Friday night, Courtney said her hello's to her Grandparents and decided to go to bed.

Later the next day, she was unable to keep fluids down, became weak, and still had that nagging little dry cough. We took her to the hospital on the next day, Saturday. After her chest films we were told she had pneumonia. Because of the extent of the pneumonia, they said they planned to admit her for two or three days. By the next morning, however, Courtney's breathing became more and more rapid and they rushed her to the ICU. Soon after that it was decided to transfer her to a much larger hospital. In spite of all that was done over the next week, Courtney's condition continued to worsen. After one week, on Saturday, July 10, 1999, Courtney was taken off life support and died within minutes.

We thank God for giving us the opportunity to parent and raise our Courtney.

There is not a day that goes by that we do not have some memory, or learn something from her writing that she left behind. She taught many of us, even in our little Cedarburg, Wisconsin community. We hear of lessons learned from many of her friends and persons we never met. They tell us of the changes they have made in their lives because of who she was and what she did in her short life.

Courtney had a dream to find a cure for all disease. We want to help her reach that goal and find a cure for ARDS. It is our mission to do everything possible to aid in reaching that goal, in helping others, whether it be fundraising for research or giving to others.

We lost our daughter after an eight-day fight with ARDS, but our fight to conquer ARDS will continue with her spirit. Courtney is truly a gift from God – for all of us!

I find myself at a loss for words when speaking to a family like Courtney's. All the usual words are clichés and it feels right to cry together and say nothing... then to come alive and laugh together again. Let us dedicate this moment to Courtney and her family, and to all the Courtneys and families everywhere who are victims of ARDS – the disease unknown to so many people.

Gregory Fleckenstein
Muskegon Music Ministries man survives ARDS 4 times

I first heard of Greg Fleckenstein when I was in ARDS rehabilitation at Harborview Hospital. I learned that he provided two free tapes of any kind of music chosen by an ARDS patient. I chose Dixieland Jazz for one tape and up-beat gospel music for the other. The tapes arrived in four days and I played them daily during my recovery. I preferred "full room volume" and other patients down the hall expressed their appreciation. The nurses, however, worried that someone might be upset and made me turn down the volume.

Since then I have been in e-mail correspondence with Greg and have chatted on an old fashioned device called the telephone. I learned that he has survived ARDS on four occasions. His first ARDS occurred at Easter 1998, four days following a minor arterial by-pass in his right leg. He was on life-support for 19 days. While on a ventilator, Greg overheard medical people saying, "He probably won't make it". Wanting him to have more positive input, his wife, Nancy, brought in a small tape player to drown out the negatives with some of his favorite music. Greg experienced the power of music, which improved his outlook and his outcome. He decided to devote his life to a music ministry.

His latest episode of ARDS occurred May 28, 2002. Because he had previously filled out a DNR form, his pulmonary physician chose not to intubate him in the face of near-death blood gases. His 28 year old son drove 250 miles to the hospital and convinced the doctor to intubate and ventilate him for a five day trial. Three days later Greg improved, was extubated, and after 12 days was actually released from the hospital.

"The power of music is universal. It crosses all boundaries – age, religion, race, " says Fleckenstein. Greg worked in local radio in the 1970's and '80's and spent 23 years as an instructor at Baker College. He uses his collection of over 2500 recordings to produce customized tapes. He encounters no copyright problems since he makes the tapes individually and gives them away at no cost.

Requests or contributions can be made to Greg's IRS 501 C(3) corporation, Muskegon Music Ministries, 1423 Moody Street, Whitehall, MI 49461. (231) 894-9395.

V CONCLUSIONS
Implications for Health Care and YOU!

1. There is a lack of awareness about ARDS.

This is the first full sized book introducing ARDS (Acute Respiratory Distress Syndrome) to the general public – and, indeed, to many physicians. ARDS can strike anyone at any age and may start with a simple cough or chest trauma.

2. There is a need for more study of survival factors for ARDS.

In spite of a mortality of between 30 - 50% advances in care have improved the outlook for individuals fortunate enough to be at a medical center with up-to-date approaches to treatment. Nevertheless, there are largely unrecognized forces BEYOND MEDICINE which appear to play a role in the survival of certain cases, such as some of those related in this book.

3. Stories have more impact than statistics in producing change.

This book presents case examples where the powers of Love, Prayer, Touch, Humor, Music and Pets play important roles in survival and recovery. Statistical studies, although difficult, are possible for each of these elements and others beyond traditional medical care.

4. Love is truly a force for healing.

Even for the unconscious patient there is a healing power of love from any source – family, friends, physicians, nurses, and anyone else caring for the person with a critical illness. As with prayer, there is no distance limitation for the force of love. Love is the single common factor in the miraculous recoveries reported in this book.

5. Prayer works – from any distance.

Independent of any specific organized religion, there is a power in prayer that affects living beings. Controlled studies of prayer have been done and more are needed, without sectarian bias.

6. Touch is an essential element of healing beyond medicine.

Even in the unconscious person, touch is received as a healing force. This includes all forms of touch: holding hands, stroking, petting, massaging, stretching, hugging, "laying on of hands" in prayer, and any form of person to person touch. Animal petting is another form of healing touch.

7. "Never say 'oops'!"

Keep all bedside comments positive, hopeful and humorous even for the comatose patient. Humor is a creative force which benefits the patient, family and caregivers. Even in the face of crisis, laughter is a positive force. Of all the senses, a sense of humor is one of the most important. "He who laughs lasts."

8. Music is an easy, often neglected, element of healing.

Whether the patient is unconscious, stuporous, or alert (and anxious) music sends a soothing, healing message. The choice of music should be tailored to each individual's specific taste. But don't forget – at times "silence is golden".

9. Pets play an important role in healing beyond medicine.

Pets can be "pesky" but still are "man's best friend". From coma to convalescence animals have been shown to be a healing force. More clinical trials are needed of pets in health care.

10. Each of us with an open mind has more to learn about healing "Beyond Medicine".

****

VI REFERENCES

The following 68 references may or may not duplicate references given in the text. They certainly do not include many books which were informative in my thinking, and include many on my "To Read" list. At least they are in alphabetical order.

Adams, P., Gesundheit!, Healing Arts Press, 1993.

Barry, D., Stay Fit and Healthy Until You're Dead, Rodale Press, 1985.

Bohm, D., "Science and Spirituality, The Need for a Change in Culture" Fetzer Institute, 1990.

Bounds, E.M., The Possibilities of Prayer, Whitaker House, 1994.

Burns, G., Dr. Burns' Prescription for Happiness, Perigee Books, 1984.

Buscaglia, L., Living, Loving, and Learning, Fawcett Columbine, 1982.

Buscaglia, L., Love, Fawcett Crest, 1972.
"A warm and wonderful book about the largest experience in life."

Canfield, J., et al, Chicken Soup for the Pet Lover's Soul, Stories about Pets as Teachers, Healers, Heroes and Friends, Health Communications, 1998.

Carlson, R. and Shield, B., editors, Healers on Healing, Penguin Putnam,1989.

Chadwick, D. and Smith, D., "The misdiagnosis of epilepsy," BMJ USA, 2: pp.245-246, May 2002.
This brief editorial from Liverpool, UK observes that syncope is the

phenomenon commonly mistaken for convulsive seizures.

Chopra, D., How to Know God, Harmony Books, 2000.

Clark and Elkinton, The Quaker Heritage in Medicine, The Boxwood Press, 1978.
Cousins, N., Anatomy of an Illness, as Perceived by the Patient, Reflections on Healing and Regeneration, Bantam Books, 1979.

Cousins, N., The Healing Heart, Avon Books, 1983.

Dalai Lama, Ethics for the New Millennium, Riverhead Books, 1999. My son, Thomas, gave this to me for Christmas following my accident and ARDS.

Dalai Lama, The Good Heart, A Buddhist Perspective on The Teachings of Jesus, Wisdom Publications, 1996.

Dossey, L., Healing Words: The Power of Prayer and the Practice of Medicine, Harpe SanFrancisco, 1993.

Dossey, L., Prayer is Good Medicine, HarperSanFrancisco, 1996.

Dossey, L., Reinventing Medicine, Beyond Mind-Body To a New Era of Healing, HarperSanFrancisco, 1999.

Fearheiley, D., Angels Among Us, Avon Books, 1993.

Foster, R., Prayers From the Heart, HarperSanFrancisco, 1994.

Frankl, Viktor, Man's Search For Meaning: An Introduction to Logotherapy, Pocket Books, 1959.

Fulgrum, R., Maybe (Maybe Not), Second Thoughts From A Secret Life, Villard Books, 1993.

Gebelein, E., Wilderness As Healer, Thornton Publishing, Inc, 2000.

Halberstam, Y. and Leventhal, J., Small Miracles, Extraordinary Coincidences from Everyday Life, Adams Media Corporations, 1997.

Hershkowitz, S., ed., Dog Tales for the Heart, Stories of Hope, Love, and Wisdom, High Impact Publications, 1995.
Jampolsky, G. and Jampolsky, L., "Listen To Me…", A book For Women and Men about Father-Son Relationships, Celestial Arts, 1996.

Jampolsky, G., Love is Letting Go of Fear, Bantam Books, 1981.

Jampolsky, G., One Person Can Make A Difference, Bantam Books, 1992.

Jantz, G., Becoming Strong Again, Fleming H. Revell, 1998.

Jaret, P., "Can Prayer Heal?", Hippocrates, pp. 31-35, April 1998.

Krantz, L., Facts! That Matter, Everything You Need To Know About Everything, Price Stern Sloan, 1993.

Lucado, M., The Greatest Moments, Word Publishing, 1995

Mandino, O., The Greatest Salesman…The Greatest Secret…The Greatest Miracle in The World, Bonanza Books, 1981.

Masson, J., Dogs Never Lie About Love, Reflections on the Emotional World of Dogs, Three Rivers Press, 1997.

McMahon, S., Carpe Diem, Seize The Day, Chronicle Books, 1995. *A little book of Latin phrases.*

Moody, R., Laugh After Laugh, The Healing Power of Humor, Headwaters Press, 1978.

Moyers, B., Healing and the Mind, Doubleday, 1993.

Myss, Caroline, Why People Don't Heal and How They Can,

Harmony Books, 1997.

Osler, W., A Way of Life, Reprinted by J. B. Lippincott, 1992.
Based on an address delivered April, 20, 1913.

Peale, N., The Power of Positive Thinking, Fawcett Columbine, 1952.

Roker, A., Don't Make Me Stop this Car! – Adventures in Fatherhood, Scribner, 2000.

Sauvage, L., The Open Heart, Stories of Hope, Healing, and Happiness, Health Communications, 1996.

Sheldrake, R., Dogs that Know When Their Owners Are Coming Home, and Other Unexplained Powers of Animals, Three Rivers Press, 1999.

Siegel, B., Love, Medicine, and Miracles, Lessons Learned From Self-Healing From A Surgeon's Experience With Exceptional Patients, Harper & Row, 1986.

Smart, Phil, Sr., Angels Among Us by The Real Santa Claus, Roots and Wings Foundation (www.roots-wings.com), Limited Edition, 2001.

Smollin, A., Tickle Your Soul, Sorin Books, 1999.

Spurgeon, C., The Power in Prayer, Whitaker House, 1996.

Steiger, B. and Steiger, S., Animal Miracles, Inspirational And Heroic True Stories, Adams Media Corporation, 1999.

Tebbetts, C., Self Hypnosis and Other Mind Expanding Techniques, Westwood Publishing, 1997.
Charles Tebbetts, one of my friends and patients, wrote this book that is one of the simplest and most practical books I have ever read on hypnosis.

Tenney, T., <u>The God Chasers</u>, Destiny Image Publishers, 1998.

Thornton, E.J., <u>Angel On Board</u>, Thornton Publishing, 1998.
www.AngelOnBoard.com

Thurber, J., and Rosen, M., ed., <u>The Dog Department, James Thurber on Hounds, Scotties, and Talking Poodles</u>, Harper Collins Publishers, 2001.

Tobin, Martin, <u>"Advances in Mechanical Ventilation,"</u> New England Journal of Medicine, pp. 1986-1996, June 28, 2001.

Turner, Dale, <u>Grateful Living</u>, High Tide Press, 1998.
This 272-page book is a collection of the weekly newspaper articles of an amazing minister and teacher.

Turner, Dale, <u>Landing Wheels</u>, The Seattle Times, 1992.

Turner, Dale, <u>Let's Think About It</u>, The Seattle Times, 1996.
Wayne, M. and Yarnall, S., The New Dr. Cookie Cookbook, Quill, 1994.

Wendell, E., Grand-Stories, <u>101+ Bridges of Love, Joining Grandparents and Grandkids</u>, Friendly Oaks Publications, 2000.
My experience being led home by my grandfather's horse when I was lost in the woods is a metaphor for letting go of the reins to be shown the way home.

Whitehead, T. and Slutsky, A., <u>"Managing the best of both old and new therapies,"</u> The Journal of Respiratory Diseases, 23: pp. 287-295, May 2002.
This is a clinical review from Toronto, including the use of lower tidal volumes, higher levels of PEEP, prone positioning, and permissive hypercapnia.

Wilkinson, B., <u>The Prayer of Jabez</u>, Multnomah Publishers, 2000.

Woodward, K., <u>The Book of Miracles, The Meaning of the Miracle</u>

Stories in Christianity, Judaism, Buddhism, Hinduism, and Islam, Simon & Schuster, 2000.

Wooten, P., Heart, Humor, and Healing, Commune-a-Key Publishing, 1994.

Wright, H. Norman, A Friend Like No Other: Life Lessons From the Dogs We Love, Harvest House Publishers, 1999.
A charming book with illustrations by Jim Lamb.

Yoder, J., Healing: Prayer or Pills?, Herald Press, 1975.

Zadra, D. and Lambert, Katie, Little Miracles, Com Pendium, Inc., 1996.
This is a delightful collection of inspiring quotes.

For more Life Enhancing books from
Thornton Publishing, Inc.
Please visit:
www.BooksToBelieveIn.com

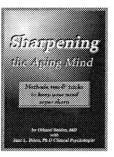

Sharpening the Aging Mind
Tools to keep your mind in tact, in shape and sharp as a tack!

Othniel J. Seiden, MD
ISBN: 0-9801941-7-2   19.97

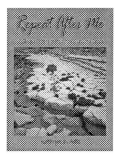

Repeat After Me
Simple Truths to Help You Survive Crisis

Kathryn D. Adis
ISBN: 0-9944838-7-X   12.97

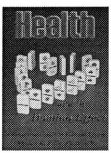

Health & the Domino Effect
A Proactive Guide to Vibrant Living through Balanced Nutrition

Sharon R. Price, Ph.D., CN
ISBN: 1-932344-55-1   19.97

To order copies of

Beyond Medicine

online at:
BooksToBelieveIn.com/BeyondMedicine.php

by phone: (303) 794-8888

by fax: (720) 863-2013

by mail:
send check payable to:

Thornton Publishing, Inc
17011 Lincoln Ave. #408
Parker, Colorado 80134

Quantity: _____ x (19.95+ 2.50 s&h) 22.45 =_____

Name: _____

Address: _____

_____

Phone: _____

E-mail _____

Credit Card #: _____

Card Type: _____   Expiration Date: ____/ ____

Signature: _____

To obtain information on having Dr Yarnall as a speaker or for a book-signing event please write, call or fax using the above information.